how to be beautiful

how to be beautiful

the thinking woman's guide

kathleen baird-murray

Vermilion
LONDON

1 3 5 7 9 10 8 6 4 2

First published 2002 by Vermilion,
an imprint of Ebury Press, Random House,
20 Vauxhall Bridge Road, London SW1V 2SA
www.randomhouse.co.uk

Random House Australia (Pty) Limited
20 Alfred Street, Milsons Point, Sydney,
New South Wales 2061, Australia

Random House New Zealand Limited
18 Poland Road, Glenfield, Auckland 10, New Zealand

Random House South Africa (Pty) Limited
Endulini, 5a Jubilee Road, Parktown 2193, South Africa

The Random House Group Limited Reg. No. 954009

Papers used by Vermilion are natural, recyclable products made from wood grown in sustainable forests.

Typeset by Palimpsest Book Production Limited,
Polmont, Stirlingshire

Printed and bound in Great Britain by
Mackays of Chatham plc, Chatham, Kent

A CIP catalogue record for this book is available from the British Library.

ISBN 0 09 188431 4

CONTENTS

For my father, who always told me I should write a book, but who sadly didn't live to see it. This probably wasn't the book you envisaged, but it's a start. And to Armand and Emmanuelle, who epitomise the true meaning of beauty.

ACKNOWLEDGEMENTS

I consider myself lucky to have had the help and support of my friends, family and close colleagues as a constant factor during the writing of this book. I have also made many new friends, who have given their time and expertise willingly and without counting the cost.

I would especially like to thank all those publicists who helped set up interviews with the experts featured in this book. They worked like a silent army and were incredibly helpful and effective without demanding anything from me in return. Debs Athey and Felicity Calthrop at Calthrop Publicity, Fiona Dowal and Owen Walker at Dowal Walker PR, the press office at Estée Lauder, Meena Khera at MKPR, Mark Smith from MRA Public Relations, Riverhouse, Kathy Djonlich from Sundari, New York and Julietta Longcroft at The Communications Store, and many others – I am hugely indebted for all your help.

There are over 40 interviews in this book – some short, some longer – with people who are at the top of their professions, as well as a few friends, and I am hugely grateful for their time and patience. This book really would not exist without the contributions of: John Barrett, Bastien, Pierre Bourdon, Lee Bradley, Nicky Clarke, Barbara Daly, Jackie Denholm Moore, Robin Derrick, Roja Dove, Malvina Fraser, John Frieda, Daniel Galvin, Peter Gray, Terry de Gunzberg, Hamilton, Lyn Harris, Robin Harvey, William Howe, the J Sisters, Philip Kingsley, Wendy Lewis, Eve Lom, Sam McKnight, Dr Daniel Maes, Jeffrey Miller, Dr Danné Montagu-King, Kay Montano, Jade Moon, Judy Naake, the Nars cosmetics make-up team, Marian Newman, Jane Oppenheim, Dr Laurie Polis, Otilyah Roberts, Linda Rose, Glauca Rossi, Eugene Souliemen, Michael van Straten, Charlotte Tilbury, Christy Turlington, Kamini Vaghela, Charles Worthington. Thank you for talking freely and unreservedly to me.

Sharing early drafts of the book with friends and colleagues and hearing their opinions was also helpful. I have bored the pants off Vassi Chamberlain, Simon Cherry, Ateh Damachi, Elise Garland, Geordie Greig, Kaja Reiff Musgrove, Caroline O'Grady, Laura Patten, Harriet Quick, Nikki Tibbles and no doubt hundreds more – thank you for listening. Thanks also go to Rosemary Scoular and Sophie Lauriemore at Peters Fraser and Dunlop for believing in the book and guiding me through every stage. Jacqueline Burns, Fiona MacIntyre, Kate Adams, Julia Kellaway, Miren Lopategui, Senate Design, Stina Smemo and Sarah Bennie at Ebury were also wonderful at putting the whole thing together and getting it out there. Jo Tutchener at Purple and Ellen Spann from Claridges have both gone way beyond the call of duty to help me – again, thank you.

There was a point where I was feeling a little despondent about the way things were going, and Richard Allan, Rebecca Anderson and my best friend Paul McNeil all put me back on the right track and told me to persevere. I cannot tell you how happy you made me just by responding directly to my little dilemma.

To my family, whose encouragement has helped me from the moment the idea was conceived to seeing it on the shelves, thank you for telling me which bits to cut, and taking the kids out for long walks so that I could write. Mummy, you probably don't remember this, but you once gave me the best beauty advice ever: don't pluck your eyebrows until you are at least 18.

And finally, special thanks to my husband Olly Daniaud, who ended up bankrolling much of this project, constantly told me that everything I wrote was brilliant even when it wasn't, and, most importantly, looked after Armand and Emmanuelle whenever I had to go away. Knowing I could rely on your support has given me the confidence I needed to finish it.

'Hi, my name is Kathleen, and
I'm a beauty editor.'

INTRODUCTION

'Shoot me if I ever write a beauty book.' That's what I used to say as one worthy book after another arrived on my desk. Full of glossy pictures, and 1001 ways to shave your legs/put on an eye cream/run a brush through your hair, the images seemed designed to tantalise, the words worthy of a quick read, but the overall effect – however pretty or clever – would invariably fall at the first fence in favour of the latest issue of *Hello!* or a chunky Margaret Atwood. Aimed at teenagers or die-hard beauty enthusiasts, they failed to pull me in, to get me excited, to teach me anything I needed to know. With a few exceptional exceptions, they were boring. Did my friends read them? No. They preferred to pick my brains over dinner, do whatever or go wherever their friends were doing or going.

And then it occurred to me. These must be the wrong books. Because the world of beauty – at least the way I see it as a 'beauty editor' – is a fascinating one. I love my job. I'm writing this as I watch the sun rise in Mexico, where I'm shooting pictures of a spa for a forthcoming issue of *Tatler* magazine. True, we've been up since 5 a.m., but we'll probably be out on a yacht today to take pictures – me and the team of photographer, models, hair and make-up, and beauty assistant. This afternoon I'll wander into the nearby town and check out some local beauty parlours for a feature I'm writing on Mexican spa traditions. Back in London I'll attend the launches of the latest anti-wrinkle miracles, the newest cosmetic colours, the next big thing in perfumes. I will be wined and dined by the heads of cosmetic corporations and public relations people. At home, I'll cleanse, tone and moisturise; shampoo, wash and perfume my body; make up my face and style my hair with products I have been asked to test, to try, to see what I think, to write about only if there is any room on any of my pages. And I know that in a small way I am shaping the face of beauty.

From my front-line vantage point I can see that in a practical, here-are-some-beauty-tips kind of fashion, we have come far in our quest to be beautiful. We have moved on from the age where a Body Shop Dewberry Bath Oil was the utmost in pampering to a more sophisticated era where the number of our local nail bar is stored in our mobile phone. Where once we dreamed of having a hair stylist or a make-up artist as our flatmate (how perfect would that be?) we now wish it were possible to have an art director for a little virtual retouching: pert breasts, smooth skin, full lips with just the flick of a pen on a screen. We are deluged with information from all angles – magazines bombard us with features on obtaining the perfect body as soon as we hit the month of March; even TV commercials throw words at us like nanospheres, liposomes, anti-hydroxy acids, and Retin-A, as if these things should be a part of our everyday vocabulary. We 'push back cuticles', we 'dry brush our skin' and 'regularly apply sun block' without ever wondering why, or whether we are doing this the right way. In fact, we're very keen on this beauty thing.

But for all that we know, we still don't always celebrate beauty for the life-enriching thing that it is. The reality of life is that beauty is often the make-or-break factor in careers, relationships, friendships. We are still judged, and judge others, according to lipstick shades – go too pink and you're silly, girly; beigey pink and you're sleek, well turned out, confident. We want to be seen to be presentable, smart, finished, but not look as if we've spent more than five minutes getting ourselves ready. We feel guilty about spending time thinking about the way we look because to do so is to spend time thinking about ourselves; to do so is to be vain, frivolous and self-indulgent, when we should probably be thinking about worthier things: world crises, tomorrow's deadline, filling the fridge. We allow ourselves the bare minimum but no more – cleanliness is next to godliness, so that's okay, but God never said anything about toning, moisturising, botoxing and finishing with a perfectly outlined lipstick'd mouth. Beauty is frippery-frappery, the whistles and bells on an already stressful, cluttered, too-busy-for-girly-nonsense kind of life. Worse still, beauty actually makes us feel uncomfortable. A young beautiful girl is often shunned by older women around her because she is a threat. She's a bimbo. And as for myself, when I tell people what I do for a living, I mumble, take a run at it, and hope they won't hear, or pronounce it with all the gusto of a recovering alcoholic on a 12-step programme: 'Hi, my name is Kathleen and I am a beauty editor.'

This book is a celebration of all that beauty is, of the people who make beauty interesting; the real experts who polish and pamper, gloss and glamorise, and who transform us from humdrum beings into the sleek, smooth creatures we are deep down. These people are so passionate about beauty that they travel the world with it, sometimes make vast amounts of money from it, and will talk the hind legs off a donkey about it. And if this still feels frivolous to you, remember that beauty, and the fantastic world it inhabits, has a therapeutic effect that goes far beyond lip gloss and liposuction. Don't believe it? Next time you have a horrible day take a long soak in a hot bath, with a glass of champagne and Clarins Beauty Flash Balm slathered all over your face.

How do you know when you've mastered the art of being beautiful? When you feel better from the outside in. When someone asks if you've been on holiday lately and you haven't. When a spritz of gardenia perfume takes you right back to the gardenia bushes on a Sydney street that you used to walk past on your way to the beach. When a tan you know you shouldn't have manages to transform all those dull old clothes at the back of your wardrobe. When you can't bring yourself to throw out a manky lipstick at the bottom of your handbag because your best girlfriend gave it to you on a drunken night out. If it makes you feel better, makes you feel you can actually do something about the way you look without feeling bad about it, then the pursuit of beauty is not such a bad thing. Because to be truly beautiful you need two things that books can't teach and money can't buy: genes and happiness. In the meantime, get plucking.

And now that I have actually gone ahead and written a beauty book – please don't shoot me.

'She's got perfect skin . . . yeah perfect skin'
Lloyd Cole and the Commotions

Chapter One

THE QUEEN OF CLEANSE

Sooner or later – and it's usually sooner – a beauty editor is confronted with a dilemma of such magnificent proportions that it throws her whole career into orbit. She spends sleepless nights tossing and turning, weeks on end reading vast tomes of pseudo-scientific beauty books, and asks – surreptiously, of course, because no one will admit to not knowing the answers – her peers, numerous experts, and the girls behind the Estée Lauder counter: Do anti-ageing creams really work?

To ask such a question is a bit like asking 'Does Jesus really exist?' or 'Is Father Christmas real?', because, disappointingly, there is no real answer beyond some scientific evidence, some testing, and a good measure of Suspension of Disbelief. No wonder they call them Hope in a Jar.

Why is it so important to know? First of all, I just hit 34 and it's starting to happen – you know, the ageing thing – and I think I should know. And secondly, it's the question people ask me as soon as they find out what I do for a living. We all want one – a moisturiser that sloughs off dead skin cells, plumps up the sagging bits, gets rid of under-eye shadows, 'diminishes fine lines', knocks off 20 years – and if you can do it for under a fiver, even better. I refuse to recommend creams to anyone who asks, first because I don't know that what works for me will work for anyone else and second because I don't have the specialist knowledge that a facialist or dermatologist will have. Third, and I am now treading on dangerous ground, I am expected, to a degree, to write about new anti-ageing products – people want to know about them. So what does that make me, if I don't know the answer? A big fat liar, that's what it makes me. And I am not 100 per cent comfortable with that.

My problem is this: I am of English extraction – okay, quarter Burmese, quarter Irish, half Scottish, but I've lived in England all my life – and I seem to have made cynicism, that underlying English quality, my forte. My sense of humour, sadly, is based on the knocking down, ripping apart, tearing asunder in-joke dig-dig ha-ha kind of humour. This is a very useful trait in journalism – if you're looking for the lie in the press release, you're more likely to discover the truth. I am sure that if he were alive, and concerned with such trivial matters as anti-ageing creams, George Bernard Shaw would agree. 'The power of accurate observation is frequently called cynicism by those who don't have it,' he once said. But somewhere along the line you have to start listening to The Experts.

The Experts – and there are lots of them – don't always agree. Of course they don't, you might argue, they're trying to push their particular product's own line of thinking. In doing so, most beauty editors are left somewhat confused and some will give up entirely on the science, or facts, as they used to be known.

Before you rush to blame the beauty editor, bear in mind that the average skincare product launch goes something like this:

Arrival: Beauty press (around 30 select glossy-magazine beauty editors) arrive in a hotel suite/conference room and are greeted with tea and breakfast. Everyone makes a pretence of eating the fruit before gorging on the croissants. The PRs tick the editors off on lists as they arrive. There are always one or two who are late and keep the rest waiting. I won't name names (because often it's me).

Lecture: This always involves a diagram showing a cross-section of the skin with all its numerous layers and hair follicles, and goodness knows what else. A doctor, of either science or dermatology, talks for rather a long time, and then two or three of the journalists ask questions, while some others make notes and most start peeking into their goody bags or wondering how they can possibly reach their deadline when they are clearly about to be trapped in this conference for most of the day.

Departure: One by one everyone shuffles out, with a few inevitable 'What was all that about?' 'I think what he meant was . . .' discussions whispered conspiratorially. Most will feature the product on a 'news' page, one or two will make a phone call to The Expert and ask him to explain once more just what he meant by 'The genes which allow the synthesis of the enzyme in the nucleus of the cell . . . part of a global concept to retrain the cells to be self-sufficient by tweaking the mechanisms that exist already so that they are reactivated . . .'

If listening to The Expert isn't muddling enough, it's nothing compared with what happens when you talk to not one, but two or three Experts. I once sat through a lecture about the skin and sun given by a highly distinguished professor (of science, not dermatology . . .) who said that it was not necessary to wear a sunscreen in Britain on a normal winter's day. As the company on whose behalf he was speaking is famous for its sunscreens, I was rather impressed by this brave stance. It had always seemed ridiculous to me to have to put on my Factor 30 when I was going to be lucky to catch so much as a glimmer of sun – possibly between jumping into the cab from outside my door and jumping out again at the office. I decided to share this with some other Experts.

The Expert's Expert is unquestionably Dr Daniel Maes, the Belgian-born Vice-President of Research and Development Worldwide at Estée Lauder. He's the one they commandeer to lecture us beauty editors every time they launch a new skincare product – if he has time, that is. He's incredibly busy, as you might expect of someone who oversees the full range of biological research and testing for all 15 of the Estée Lauder brands (which include M.A.C., Clinique and Bobbi Brown to name but a few). He must be pretty good at it if Lauder's net sales of $4.4 billion in 2000 and yearly annual sales increases are anything to go by. He insists that all quotes are double-checked with him, ostensibly on the grounds of scientific accuracy, but also, one suspects, because of a certain paranoia, as the brand is famously aware of the power of marketing and the press.

Notwithstanding any reticence, we tackle the confusing issue of sunscreen.

'I was at a skincare launch a while back,' I say, 'and they said you didn't need to use sunscreen in this climate on a normal day. I was quite amazed because this particular company has always really pushed their sunscreens.'

'When you see how fast skin cancer can start, you know you are going to have to wear a sunscreen every day,' he replies, not impressed – perhaps even a little bored (to be fair, he does have a Masters in nuclear chemistry, so he'd probably rather be splitting atoms than talking about sunscreen). 'And now that we make a sunscreen that is non-irritating, I think it's a good idea to use it. But it has to be complemented by antioxidants or anti-inflammatories because sunscreen only keeps out UV light. All the smoke, pollution and ozone which we are all exposed to, those elements are controlled not just by sunscreens but by antioxidants.'

You see!

Next up: Dr Danné Montagu-King, an American Doctor of Science with a permanent tan and what looks like black eyeliner rimming his lower lids. He's definitely a smaller fish in a big pond, but he has a nice line in face peels and anti-cellulite treatments (the latter of which, incidentally, do work, albeit temporarily – I sent someone along to try them out) and a reputation for being forthright and outspoken. He should be able to give me a concise, direct answer, I think to myself.

'Do you think people should wear sunblock every day?' I say.

'Yes, but not in this weather,' he replies.

'I recently heard of a skincare company that has always been very pro-sun block, but they have now said you do not need to wear one every day.'

'Firstly, I don't agree with mixing SPF with creams and things . . . We do an SPF30 – anything more is redundant, and anything less is not good enough, simply because of the ozone layer. We will change – by 2500 everyone will have dark skin on this planet, because the human race does adapt to ecological change. It will take several generations to do this, so we are the suffering generation. Secondly, on a day when there is any type of sun at all, people should have a block, but obviously not in Britain's weather . . .'

There is no such thing as a simple answer.

So you then decide to do a little of your own research. You try the anti-ageing creams yourself. But it's very hard to see the kind of astounding results they claim. How do you know your improved skin texture isn't to do with the fact that you've had more sleep in the last couple of weeks? Or drunk more water? And what's good for your skin type might not be good for someone else's. So you find someone whose skin it suits: your mother, your mother-in-law, your boss's wife (always a good move) and ask them to test it. But you never quite know whether they're using it properly, or at all. My mother kept asking me if I had any moisturisers I could give her. 'But I've given you loads already. What on earth are you doing with them?' It turns out that the anti-ageing creams I'd given her had been stored carefully away, untouched, because I'd terrified her by telling her how powerful they are these days and that she might have to wear a sunscreen on top. She now wanted something with as much sophistication as a tub of aqueous cream.

My mother-in-law triumphantly announced that she had two firm favourites – Crème de la Mer, the super-expensive (though actually not any more, in comparison with just about every other beauty company which has since brought out moisturisers in the £150 a pot range) cream that claims to have amazing powers, thanks to its production methods (it likes to listen to a recording of the bubbling sound made by the previous batch while it in turn is being made. I kid you not.) Her second favourite was a Paloma Picasso moisturiser. 'But that's for the body!' I said. 'I don't care. It's fantastic! It smells really gorgeous!' she replied. 'Isn't it too perfumed for your face? Why don't you use it on your body?' 'Not at all! And it comes in a big tub and lasts for ages!'

I have faith in the big skincare companies because the research they do now is second to none. Most will link up with universities, which are happy to provide information in return for the huge grants they receive from the industry. It is now also very hard to make a false claim about a product thanks to the US Food and Drugs Administration (FDA), which ensures that everything on sale in the USA is for the public (hence the tag, 'FDA approved', which is often mistakenly assumed to mean that the product works, whereas it just means it's safe), and to the British Advertising Standards Authority (ASA), which responds to public complaints about products not living up to the claims made about them in magazine and newspaper advertisements. If you check out the website for the ASA, and look under 'adjudication', you will find some fascinating reading. Several 'big name' beauty brands have been forced to change the claims they make in advertising on the grounds that an independent assessor (often a dermatologist based at a university) has looked at their evidence and doesn't believe it. Any member of the public can buy a product, and if they don't believe it is doing what it claims to do in its advertising (not the packaging, over which the ASA has no authority whatsoever), they can complain and it will be investigated.

'I think there's a healthy dose of scepticism amongst the female population,' says Donna Mitchell of the ASA. 'There has to be – what advertiser is going to talk about their products in a negative way? The ASA has made decisions in the past about claims, and it does mean that companies do know how far they can go. Readers are very sophisticated now.' The very positive flip-side of this is that the consumer wields a lot of power – unless a complaint has been lodged about a particular product's advertising, you can assume that the claims you read about anti-ageing products in the advertisements can be substantiated. And if you try the product, and you don't think it works, pick up the phone and initiate an investigation.

So much scrutiny can be frustrating for The Experts. Off the record, one, who cannot be named for legal reasons, even told me he has almost given up doing press in the USA because he feels so restricted by the possibility of competitors challenging his claims, just to cause the company the inconvenience of having to prove its claims publicly.

Dr Danné Montagu-King thinks that over-the-counter skincare products may even be held back too far by such bodies. 'There are such rigorous checks now,' he says, 'you only have to look at the insurance companies and law firms in the US and see how it all begins. America is a really litigious country, and that is why they don't have a law that really affects things for over-the-counter sales. For example, sometimes when you are changing or revising a bad skin condition, there is an uncomfortable period you go through. People love to say, "I'm breaking out! I'm suing!" As a result, the skincare companies don't really want to rock any boats. The FDA doesn't care whether ingredients are effective or not, they just care if it is safe. Anything that falls under the EU laws is much more stringent than the FDA.' The ASA's line is that if a cream causes real physiological changes to the skin, i.e. wrinkles are removed *permanently*, then it's not skincare, it's medicine, and that means it needs a licence.

But the problem doesn't stop at advertising – there is nothing to stop journalists from writing whatever they like about a product. 'Editorial is more persuasive,' says Donna Mitchell. 'And if a celebrity is endorsing something, it is taken as gospel.' She's right. Who hasn't bought a tub of cream on no greater grounds than that Gwyneth Paltrow/Madonna/Jennifer Lopez has bought it? If she looks that good on it, it can't be bad, right?

But maybe it's our own wishful thinking that is to blame. The biggest misconception about anti-ageing creams is the term 'anti-ageing'. When you actually read the claims, the most they will say is that they will 'temporarily remove fine lines' or 'diminish the appearance of fine lines'. Many ordinary moisturisers will puff up the skin temporarily enough to 'diminish the appearance of fine lines', so to prove that they are more effective than ordinary moisturisers, many anti-ageing creams will have undergone comparative testing. In other words, they will improve skin texture more than most, but they don't actually claim to remove wrinkles for ever – it's we who assume this because we're paying a lot of money – sometimes up to £250 for some of the more expensive creams – and because the picture of the cream on the page is often placed next to a model whose lines, if she had any to begin with, have been cleverly retouched away. The cream *must* be a wrinkle miracle – surely?

What should you look for in an over-the-counter anti-ageing cream?

Dr Daniel Maes suggests the following: 'The basic thing is to protect your skin. Look for a moisturiser with a sunscreen, antioxidants and anti-inflammatory ingredients. When you start to notice some damage on your skin, like lines, wrinkles, age spots, then you need to use products which include some repair benefits, products that will help boost the collagen production so you can repair the damage already caused.'

SKINOLOGY – WHAT IT'S ALL ABOUT

INGREDIENTS: The following terms are bandied about with such ease that it's easy to assume we know what they mean. Just in case . . .

Anti-inflammatory agents: There are natural anti-inflammatories such as chamomile and tea tree oil, as well as more powerful steroid creams (hydrocortisones) and newer non-steroidal anti-inflammatory agents such as Protopic cream. The natural agents work by unknown mechanisms; the steroids work by 'telling' the inflammatory cells to leave the skin and go back to the bloodstream and also constrict cutaneous blood vessels; and the Protopic cream is an immunomodulator which instructs the body's overactive inflammatory cells to calm down.

Alpha hydroxy acids (AHAs): Found naturally in sugar-cane, apples, grapes, milk and olives, AHAs speed up the skin's natural exfoliation process by dissolving the dead, flaking layer of the epidermis (outer skin) and exposing the smoother, fresher skin underneath. One of these AHAs, glycolic acid is widely used because it has a small molecular structure and so can penetrate the skin easily. AHAs will leave your complexion glowing, but you may suffer from stinging or burning and increased sensitivity.

Antioxidants: These are intended to prevent the chemical reactions with oxygen that cause cell breakdown. Vitamins A, C, E, grapeseed, pomegranates, green tea and white tea are some examples of antioxidants.

Vitamin A: Also known as retinoic acid, this occurs naturally in fish, liver and oil. It makes the outer layer of the skin a little thinner, the pores smaller, and helps correct elastic tissue damage in deeper layers of skin by increasing collagen production. Retinol, Retin-A and Renova are the brand names of retinoic acid. Strong versions of vitamin A are used a lot in acne and anti-ageing creams. These are usually available on prescription.

Vitamin E: Also known as D-Alpha Tocopherol, this antioxidant is said to reduce fine lines and moisturise the skin by encouraging moisture to be absorbed upwards from the deeper layers of the skin to the epidermis.

Vitamin C: Also known as ascorbic acid, this is naturally found in rose hips and oranges. As an antioxidant, it can help to increase collagen production and destroy free radicals. It doesn't stay fresh for very long, but skincare companies have discovered some nifty ways of keeping it active for longer, including some preparations you actually mix yourself.

Promises, promises . . . but will we believe them?

Robin Harvey, a creative director at Label, the offshoot of the London-based ad agency J. Walter Thompson, thinks the advertising trend for making seemingly outrageous claims on behalf of anti-ageing creams may be on its way out. 'The more claims advertisers make, the less likely people are to believe them. First the creams had 68 per cent moisture, then it was 70 per cent. It's all very 1980s. Now almost every brief I get starts with beauty being about the individual, about beauty coming from within . . .'

If they can do such amazing things with face creams, why can't they cure skin cancer?

'Science is something which moves in very tiny steps. When we do carry out this research on the effects of energy on the cellular protection system we are indeed improving our understanding of the processes leading to cancer,' says Dr Daniel Maes. 'But cancer is a huge thing which has many other steps involved. There is a gene called P53 which is a very important gene because it decides if a cell is too damaged

to be repaired, to avoid the replication of an abnormal genetic cell. We have a research programme in Belgium where we try to understand the processes leading to cancer. We are going to ask if energy is allowing the cell to make the right decision and to eliminate the cells which are dangerous. Everyone is working on curing cancer. We are working on skin beauty, skin ageing, so indirectly skin cancer. We are using molecules which are used to prevent cancer. Green tea is an element that has been shown in Japan to prevent cancer. One scientist has extracted and improved the green tea to create a highly concentrated blend, and that blend of this molecule is now being tested as a drug to prevent topical cancer. All research is inter-twined . . . ageing, cancer, beauty. For me beauty is in the science. Just make sure the cells are healthy and from there beauty will come.'

And now, just when you almost started to believe in anti-ageing creams, Dr Danné Montagu-King says, 'NINETY-FIVE PER CENT OF THE BEAUTY INDUSTRY IS FAKE AND ANYONE CAN CHALLENGE ME ON IT.'

Hmmm. If that is the case, Dr Danné, what are we humble consumers supposed to look for in the beauty salon?

'If you go somewhere and they start touting their treatments, you have a right to ask how everything works at cellular level,' he says. 'If they cannot explain it in logical terms that you understand, walk out of the door and never come back. They have not been educated properly in anatomy, chemistry, physiology and are not using the right tools. You will be surprised how some doctors will even forget the basics and become little puppets of the drug companies.'

PROBLEM
You're suspicious of anything sold in a shop.
SOLUTION
Make it yourself.

Here are some basic kitchen-sink recipes for face-masks.

For dry skin: Mix egg yolk with a teaspoon of honey, a teaspoon of mayonnaise and a tablespoon of buttermilk. Apply to the face and leave for 20 minutes. Rinse with warm water.

For oily skin: Mix kaolin or Fuller's Earth (you can buy this from a chemist) with water. Add 1–2 drops of an essential oil such as lavender, which has natural healing and relaxing properties, and 2 tablespoons of apple cider vinegar. Apply and leave on for 20 minutes. The mask will help remove excess oil as well as drawing out any congestion from the skin. It's not suitable for sensitive skins.

For normal or combination skins: Mix half a tablespoon of fine oatmeal with a teaspoon of honey and a little warm water. Leave it on the face for 30 minutes and then massage in small circular movements for an exfoliating effect. Rinse with warm water. This mask is great for toning and tightening the complexion.

For sensitive skins: Mash 1 tablespoon of ripe avocado flesh with a few drops of almond oil, or a vitamin E capsule for a greater moisturising effect if you have dry skin. Massage it lightly into the face and leave for 30 minutes. Tissue off and rinse with lukewarm water.

What would the trendsetters like to 'fix' with the beauty industry?

Jeffrey Miller has been dubbed a 'coolhunter' by the media because he spots the next big trends and advises people how to make the most of them. Based in New York, he can re-invent the tired images of yesterday's fashion and beauty brands and turn them into desirable commodities once more. He is a passionate convert to pure and simple beauty, having been inspired by his travels to faraway places – all in the search of peoples and products that are untainted by pollution, money and celebrity values. Interestingly, he doesn't think the pressure to look young is the main problem with the beauty industry, but . . . 'The most grievous, the most unconscionable, disingenuous, crooked and unregulated promise of the past five years is not that you will be young and flawless and thin and simply beautiful, but that you will be healthy,' he says.

Miller wants the beauty industry to clean up its act, to remove chemicals from products that aren't particularly destructive or dangerous, but that might pollute the environment or be unnecessary for our skin. 'If I am to be specific,' he says, 'I would like to have my own line of products, or just go around removing one additive, a huge pet peeve, called sodium laurel sulfate, or sodium laureth sulfate, from the market place. Get it OUT of shampoos and soap and toothpaste, shaving cream, bubble bath . . . It's hideously toxic and is only there to add suds, foam, lustre, whatever the marketers in the 1950s thought would make things more appealing. Let me at this project!'

Eve Lom fixes the faces of famous people. She is a facialist. She practically invented facials. And though she is modest about her work ('A facial is only about five per cent of having good skin'), there are hundreds of models and famous faces who will happily sing her praises, including Erin O'Connor, Madonna, Cate Blanchett, Meg Ryan and Gwyneth Paltrow. Of course, it's not just famous faces she'll fix – she has been known to gently ask waitresses, shop attendants, and anyone she meets who she feels could benefit from her magic hands to come to her clinic, try a treatment, and just see what some plain, old-fashioned skincare can do.

Plain, old-fashioned skincare can restore your faith, that's for sure. I firmly believe that you can do a lot to ward off the effects of ageing with basic maintenance. One of Eve's facials makes your skin glow, leaves it looking like it can breathe, it's soft to the touch, it's all the things you ever wanted it to be. Her own skin is crystal-clear, haloed by a mane of long blonde hair tied back in a slick pony-tail. She cannot help but radiate health, strength and vitality. I suspect she is in her mid-fifties, although she will only admit to being 'as old as a good bottle of wine', and she certainly looks a lot younger. Her manner is authoritative, doubly so because when you meet her at her clinic she is invariably clad in a clean white overall. She speaks crisply, her accent pure Eastern European – she hails from Czechoslovakia where she was once a dancer.

Her facials are neither the conventional squeeze and steam approach (although she will scrub as she doesn't believe in waiting for creams to dissolve blackheads), nor the more gimmicky blast of oxygen and some weird ingredients aproach. You certainly won't get much in the way of smalltalk (thank goodness). Before she gets to work on your face, she has one of her assistants 'prep' your skin, with a deep cleanse followed by hot paraffin painted on to soften the skin. When she finally enters the room, you are aware only of a different presence. You're nearly asleep for a start, and she slips in quietly, standing behind you, and gets to work on your face, performing the lymph massage and acupressure techniques for which she is so famous.

Afterwards she will just as likely tell you you need to start doing Pilates to correct your posture as she will tell you what moisturiser to use, such is her belief in a holistic approach to skincare. She can be firm and bossy, gentle and funny. Once, just as I was leaving after a facial, she gave me a good telling off about my apparently wonky left shoulder. 'You can come back and see me again,' she said. Then, with a twinkle in her eye: 'I don't let everyone come back.' When I finally met up to interview her for this book, it was no surprise that instead of talking about cleanse, tone and moisturise, our conversation took more of a holistic bent.

It was winter, it was late. Eve had been working all day and was now waiting for the arrival of her sister from Vienna. Her phone kept ringing, so it was a while before we could talk properly. I was a little tired too, and by the end of our interview, just one hour later, we were both ready to move on, though both too polite to say. Eve seemed a little impatient, a little fierce, and I could understand how she has a reputation for not suffering fools gladly as she launched into a tirade about women who pay obscene amounts of money for anti-ageing creams:

'The world has gone bananas,' she says. 'Bananas! Women pay these prices because their pockets are being manipulated – it serves them right. If they had to plead with their husbands for an allowance of £90 to buy a moisturiser, maybe the world would still be a better place. I am old-fashioned, but what has been happening to us is that we are all brainwashed with no common sense any more. Does anyone stop and question any more? No!'

There is more. 'Most of the women I know, even though I love them, they need a bit of telling off. They are lazy, and they expect miracles. They are independent and think that if they can pay for something they can have it.'

But beneath the ferocity of her argument lies logic, plain and simple. The reason anti-ageing creams, and skincare generally, will never completely satisfy our desires to look better, younger, more glamorous, to have perfect skin and perfect lives, is because there is so much more to good skin than something you buy in a jar. Eve thinks there is no point in taking anything less than an entirely holistic approach. And she means holistic.

'It's a question of what their profession is,' she says of her clients. 'What their marital status is, what they eat, how they eat. How much water do they drink? Do they do any sport? Do they have time for themselves? How are their periods? Do they take supplements?'

She cites as an example patients of hers who had acne as teenagers. In some cases they were prescribed antibiotics for years, which left their abdominal system very vulnerable to yeast and sugar. Too much of these are known to deplete the intestinal flora, leaving the digestive system more sensitive to yeast. If their diet now consists of a lot of bread and sandwiches, they are more likely to feel bloated and constipated, and if their system is sluggish as a result, their skin is more likely to be clogged and congested.

Yet none of these things in themselves constitute 'problem' skin.

'There is no such thing,' she argues. 'Everyone at some point in their life or monthly cycle has skin that can change in 48 hours, if not quicker. You have good days and bad days. The other day someone called and asked whether I can give them a secret quick fix to have great skin before a party. I told her, 'Please don't insult me! Just take a brown bag and put it over your head.' There is no quick fix for good skin, unless you have good genes and don't abuse the skin, in which case you are lucky. And even if you are *lucky*, you have to take care of it.'

Her philosophy is very simple. The most important thing we can do for our skin, is to 'Cleanse, cleanse and cleanse!' she says. 'I am called the Queen of Cleanse. Exfoliation is extremely important. At a gentle level it is more beneficial than anti-wrinkle creams.' Her routine, which she prescribes for nearly all her clients, is to take a muslin cloth and cleanse the skin with her own brand wax-like paste, applying the cloth first hot, and then with cold water, at the same time massaging the pressure points on the face. This gentle, but daily exfoliation ensures that any dry skin that is deposited in wrinkles is removed. The overall result is younger-looking, fresher feeling skin.

'Have you always had beautiful skin?' I ask, looking at her end-of-the-day, devoid-of-make-up, perfect complexion.

'No. Yet again . . . ' and she sounds almost exasperated at this point, 'what is beautiful skin, and what is this, and what is that?!' She smiles. 'I get spots. I had four days in Paris and was eating this, that and the other. I had pig's trotter, and pâté, and champagne. I had a huge spot, which was very painful and people were like, 'Thank God! She has a spot! She is human!'

How can she possibly be so secure about her looks, her life, I wonder? As if she can read my mind (I don't know, maybe she can), she answers: 'If I am secure, it is because I have based my values on different things and not on beauty. It is a contradiction I know because I am in this business, but I am in it on a physical level. I know I can scrub my face, I can squeeze the whiteheads, and not get into the whole palaver of the propaganda.'

'You believe in maintaining skin, and keeping things simple,' I say. 'But it's not that simple, because your routine does require some effort. My mother's generation, on the other hand . . . my mother has lovely skin and has never done anything to it. She is in her sixties now, part Irish and part Burmese. Why is her skin so perfect?' (I don't dare tell her that my mother's idea of cleansing is splashing her face with soap and water – and that's it.)

'The world is a different place now,' says Eve. 'The rate of pollution has increased. The time when your mother lived and did not use anything . . . did she have the type of life we are coping with now?'

'She had big stresses . . . like war.'

'Natural life and stress,' says Eve. 'War is not natural, but family stress . . . day-to-day stress . . . Everybody is asking a fortune for everything and no one is competent in anything. Everything is artificially made. There is no time for nurturing because everything is unnatural and we are going against nature. The terrible waste! The terrible waste – not just in the way you throw things away, but the way food is packaged . . . it is actually frightening.'

'But how does stress directly affect the skin?'

'It is not so much that stress affects the skin, but it affects your body and your breathing. The circulation in the body is affected, and the brain doesn't think rationally when it is stressed out . . . Look, everything is so fragile, whether it is happiness or beauty. Nothing is static in this world, and you should just accept that. Keep a relatively even keel and you have won.'

Part of Eve's facial includes concentrating on breathing. This, she explains, is to improve the circulation and counterbalance the effects of stress. She continues: 'When you are stressed, you go on Prozac, it makes you numb and you don't respond to anything. When you are stressed you skip everything and don't wash your face. If you are anxious, you either hold your stress in your abdomen, heart, digestive system or your brain. If you hold it in your heart you will get a heart attack. We all have vulnerable points in our bodies. If you don't do anything about stress your body starts screaming for help and will pay you back. It's as if you are locking things up in a cupboard, but the cupboard needs an airing from time to time. There's no point in going to the gym if you don't breathe deeply there, as you only produce more toxins. By stressing the muscles more you are producing lactic acid.'

So we must breathe. Well, that's fine, I can do that. In, out – look, no hands!

'*Shallow* breathing! Women do not fill their bodies and do not have a clue! They beat up their bodies in the day and then again at night in the gym, and the mind is not there.'

Later, a few weeks later, I think about what stress is doing to us all. My sister tells me how a day at home, waiting for engineers to come and fix something, almost drove her to tears of frustration. I think about a male friend of mine who breaks out in the fiercest rash from head to toe for no apparent reason. And I'm not proud of it, but I did lose my temper recently so spectacularly in a French airport that I was nearly arrested, although these days it's actually very easy to get arrested at an airport – there are signs telling you how easy it is all over the place. I think about the collective stress a city like New York must have suffered when the Twin Towers came down. Of how we're all seeing and dealing with things our parents would never have imagined we would be dealing with. And in spite of all this stress, what do we choose to actually worry about? Wrinkles.

Why can hot and cold be good for the face?

Eve's system of cleansing alternates a hot cleansing cloth with a cold one. Heat can speed up the healing process, particularly if it is followed with cold. The combination will speed up a sluggish circulation and bring the blood up quickly to the surface of the skin, allowing the white blood cells to ingest any infection and reduce inflammation. Use the warm water first, to open the pores and allow your cleanser to have the greatest effect, then follow with cold water to close them. This is a method that calls for a degree of common sense – if you apply too much heat and too much cold you are likely to cause the delicate facial blood vessels to break.

What should a professional facial do for your skin?

The bottom line is that you should feel you have achieved more effective deep cleansing than you can do yourself. Most will offer a proper extraction process that will remove any blackheads or whiteheads but not leave the skin looking and feeling damaged. They will include either a lymph drainage or deep tissue massage that will reduce the puffiness of the skin and drain the toxins and excess fluid. At some point, heat may be used, either in the way of a heated mask, or by steam. If you suffer from rosacea, steam should be avoided – a good therapist will know how much heat any skin type can take.

How can you find a good facialist?

A word of mouth recommendation by someone you trust is the best way. When you call up, find out what the facial actually entails. Ask a few questions. The environment should always be clean, as should the therapist. They should be able to tell just by looking and touching your skin what the problem is, and should be able to advise you what the best course of action is. Alternatively, call skincare companies such as Darphin, Decleor, or Clarins to find out who is good in your area.

How can you give yourself a facial at home?

Use a normal cream cleanser to remove your make-up. With a soft brush (try goat's hair, or even a soft shaving brush) go over the skin with a foaming cleanser and a little water to help clarify the pores. Use an exfoliating product – they work by sticking to the dead skin cells and gently peeling them off. (At this point, you'll probably be contemplating a good squeeze of your spots – but don't even think about it. Spot squeezing is only for the brave, the foolish, and professional facialists.) Put on a face mask for your skin type for ten minutes or so, then remove. (If your skin is dry, you'll need something that is hydrating, if it is clogged, something that is deep cleansing, etc.) Take a muslin cloth and soak it in warm water. Put a couple of drops of lavender oil on the cloth and wrap it over your face while still warm. Follow with a face massage using an oil that is suitable for the face and two soft sable brushes to brush upwards in a light, circular motion, avoiding the eye area. Massage gets the circulation moving, helps with congestion, and is great for puffiness.

Eve Lom wishes we wouldn't . . .

Neglect ourselves. 'Hands, feet and face. Not paying attention to your children, bank account and profession, it is all the same thing. Do not expect your flowers to grow if you neglect to water them. All I try and do is to minimise the work of the face, and I think I have succeeded rather well. I am impatient and don't have time to fiddle. When I travel, I have three pots in my bag.'

Diet – what can it do for the skin?

Eve's holistic approach means that sooner or later we have to take into account what we eat and drink. Most of us have a balanced diet – unless we're seduced by the lure of the quick-fix detox, in which case a multi-vitamin supplement may be necessary. What you're eating won't cause acne, but bingeing on one kind of food over another may not leave your skin at its best. Avoid excessive amounts of alcohol and caffeine. Drink lots of water alongside any alcohol. Laxatives and diuretics used over a long period are not just bad for your whole system but will also affect your skin. If you have very dry skin this can sometimes indicate a deficiency in vitamin A, in which case take a cod liver oil supplement, or try to eat more fish, liver and milk. Oily skin can sometimes be due to a lack of vitamin B2 or B6. Stock up on fresh fruit and vegetables – in particular asparagus, blueberries, broccoli, cantaloupe melon, carrots, red peppers, tomatoes, sweet potatoes, oranges, avocados, wholewheat bread, chicken, milk, tea and seafood. These are especially good sources of antioxidants, vitamins and minerals. And be sure to drink lots of water.

Is sunscreen the best protection against ageing?

'Most of my life I have been a rebel,' says Eve. 'What is a sunblock for? It is a multi-million-dollar industry. Why would I put sunblock on when I am going to sit in the shade? Why do I need a sunblock when I walk into the office at 8.30 a.m. and leave at 6.30 p.m.? When I go swimming, that's when I'll put sunblock on. In the summer between 11 a.m. and 3 p.m. I won't sit in the sun. But I love walking in the warm sun. When we're stuck inside with central heating . . . no one will tell me sun is bad for me.'

And if you can't find that paper bag to put over your face before a party . . . *an old party-trick is to apply a mask of whisked egg white with a few drops of lemon juice to tighten the skin before you go out. Leave it to harden, and then rinse with warm water.*

And then it happened. Suddenly I had something new to worry about. From nowhere, and as if by magic, although this is no magic you'd want to bring into your life, tiny, red, bumpy, itchy spots appeared behind my ears. At first they were a curiosity – like a pet biology project that I could cultivate. 'Look at what happens if I scratch!' But the more I scratched, the more they spread, downwards towards my neck, inching along, all the time itching and burning, hotter and hotter, until it was all I could do not to touch them. 'Can you see anything behind my ears?' I asked my husband. He put down our son and came to the bathroom where the light was brighter for a close-up examination. 'Yuk! Ugh! That's revolting!' he said. A scream, echoing my husband's, came from the other room, causing us to abort our inspection, as our son seized upon the opportunity of being left alone in a room with his little sister to wallop her on the head. Later, when I had my husband's full and undivided attention, he administered antiseptic. 'You have to see a specialist,' he said.

Have you ever tried getting an appointment with a specialist, in this case a dermatologist? I couldn't even get an appointment at my local doctor's for a referral to a dermatologist. I settled for the advice of my local pharmacist, who told me I was experiencing an allergic reaction to something I had used on my skin, or even a pair of earrings, or shampoo. He gave me an anti-histamine tablet to stop the itching, and a range of skincare for sensitive skins that I was to use for three weeks.

How did I feel about this? Special! At last I had joined the elite ranks of those with allergies, those sensitive skin people who can't eat this, drink that, use this, or breathe that. And then I found it extremely annoying. That favourite moisturiser? Out of bounds. My new face mask? Strictly forbidden. And in the meantime, tying my hair back so it wouldn't irritate the hideous spots was really not a good look – now they were on display for the whole world to see.

They went away, of course, after about three days, although I bragged about them for much longer. Nonetheless, I thought it typical that it was something I was only interested in when I suffered from it myself.

According to facialist Jackie Denholm Moore – another old-school professional who has the dubious privilege of tending to my skin on occasion – sensitive skin can take many forms. 'There's touch sensitive skin, which is the sort of skin that when you touch it, it comes up all blotchy. People with touch-sensitive skin tend to get rashes when they're worried or a little stressed about something – you press the skin and it comes up instantly red.'

'That's not mine,' I say.

'The other types of sensitive skin are reactive sensitive – for example, they are sensitive to lanolin, and should only use things that are hypoallergenic or unperfumed. You can get skin like this by using products that are too aggressive. The skin needs to protect itself more, so it develops an extra protection method, which causes it to become extra sensitive. But pollution can also trigger it, as can sun exposure, hard water . . . And if you have thin skin it can be even more delicate.'

I probably receive about 30 different skincare products a week, sent to me to try out. My bathroom cabinet is full to the brim of expensive and inexpensive creams. I have something for everything: face masks to pick me up and put me down; moisturisers for when my skin is dry, dehydrated, oily, normal, or all of these things at once. I have serums, for I still don't know what. I have eye creams and eye oils; face creams and face oils. I have spot creams and sensitive skin creams. Creams that will plump out wrinkles, or brighten my face. Natural creams, and creams packed full of the latest technological advances and miracle ingredients. I try them out whenever feasibly possible. I probably embark on a different routine every three days. A dermatologist once told me that the average number of foreign ingredients women expose their skin to via cosmetic preparations on an average day is something like 40 to 60. It would be more surprising if you didn't react to anything. Trying to establish what it was that caused my rash was going to be impossible.

Denholm Moore's advice was no more exciting than the pharmacist's. I was going to have to give up using water on my face, at least for a while, and use gentle, soothing, calming products. 'Nothing that's harsh, nothing that will strip the skin, nothing aggressive,' she says. 'Treat it gently, and when you're cleansing don't rub too hard.'

Perfumes were to be avoided, especially synthetic ones. Eve Lom had also warned about these: 'The worst place to wear them is behind the ear because all the lymph glands are there, and if you have a tendency to oily skin you can be sure you will get a spot there.'

The spots behind my ears led me to think about spots generally. What about those really big ones that rear their ugly head(s) from time to time, demanding to be picked and prodded, coaxed from their warm, comfortable beds and out into the big, bad world of cotton wool and antiseptic? Blackheads, whiteheads, or those huge carbuncles? What about them? What about acne? There is so much more to worry about than wrinkles!

Denholm Moore is a little calmer than myself. She takes each of these problems on board and deals with them thoughtfully, yet matter of factly. And this is what she says:

'If you just can't leave your spots alone, take a muslin cloth and warm up the skin, making sure it is scrupulously clean. Take 2 tissues, double them up, and wrap them around your fingers. With the index finger, squeeze down and up, so you're not actually using your nails, but just the pads of your fingers. If the spot won't do anything, leave it alone, but if it comes out fairly easily, put some toner on the area you've extracted to tighten up the pores, then put some tea tree oil on a cotton bud and dab it on the area. Then put a mask on – preferably a deep cleansing one – to draw it out like a poultice. When you've removed that, put a muslin over the area you have just extracted, only this time apply it really cold, after running it under the cold tap. Don't put on any make-up afterwards, just go to bed and let it run its course.'

'But what if there's still something nasty lurking there?'

'Take some cotton wool, run it under a hot, but not scalding tap, and hold the hot cotton wool over the area. Then quickly get your tissues again and squeeze down and up. Normally when you squeeze a spot, if it's one of those nasty ones, you will get a tiny spot of blood that means it's all out. You can usually tell. If it's been throbbing, it will instantly go as soon as it's out. But you must remember the mask and the tea tree oil.'

I should tell you, Jackie Denholm Moore was extremely reluctant to tell me how to squeeze spots. She really thinks you should leave it to a professional. You'll know if you've gone too far because the skin will look browner afterwards – this is a sign that you have damaged the skin. Of course, it's not much comfort to know that after the fact, is it?

MORE SKINOLOGY

WHAT DOES IT ALL MEAN?

Hypoallergenic: This means there should be no product in a cream that is reactive to skin, such as menthol, lanolin, peppermint or anything that might aggravate.

Non-comedogenic: This is usually found on packaging to describe a product that has ingredients that won't clog up the skins and give you blackheads. Some balmy or waxy ingredients that are fantastic for a dry or dehydrated skin are not so good for skin that congests easily because they cause a film to form under the skin that can block the pores.

1001 REALLY BAD SPOTS: ADVICE FROM JACKIE DENHOLM MOORE

If you have *spots everywhere* and can't stop squeezing them, go to the doctor and get an antiobiotic topical solution to dab on and kill off any infection you might have caused through touching them too much. This is a problem young girls often have. Keep on applying a deep cleansing mask to draw the spots to the surface and get them out, rather than squeezing them. A purifying mask that doesn't harden can be applied to the spot overnight, which will stop you from picking it.

Blackheads are a build-up of dead skin, oil and rubbish from underneath that gets blocked in the pore. When it hits the surface of the skin, it is oxidised by the air, and this turns it black. Occasionally you'll get them in your cheeks if you haven't cleansed properly, and sometimes they'll turn into spots because they get irritated underneath, but usually you get them around the nose and chin areas and wherever you have excess oil. Exfoliating and using a face mask once a week will really help, as will going to have a facial every two months. If you can't do this, just ask for a steam, a cleanse and a face mask.

Carbuncles feel like a huge lump underneath the skin. They tend to occur on either side of the chin, and are usually hormonal. Never squeeze them. Skin brush for lymph drainage, apply a spot solution or tea tree oil regularly, apply deep-cleansing masks up to three times a week just on that spot, and eventually they will go away. Be warned, they can take up to three weeks to disappear.

Whiteheads, or milia, are sometimes caused by dryness, but they can also be acid spots, from when you have eaten too many spicy foods or tomatoes, or drunk too much white wine. They are tiny, hard white lumps which form underneath the skin and look like pin pricks. You must NEVER remove these by yourself – a professional will do it with a sterile needle.

Acne: I thought this only happened to teenagers . . . You thought wrong. *Acne vulgaris* is the big lumpy, weepy kind that tends to come with teenage skins, but can also affect adults. *Acne rosacea* is broken veins and high colouring, with spots mixed in, and is also affected by heat. I e-mailed my new best friend, New York dermatologist Dr Laurie Polis (who you'll hear a lot more from in the next chapter), because really, if you have acne, or think you might have, you should see a dermatologist, as any good facialist will tell you. 'Causes of acne in adults mostly include genetics, hormones and some environmental factors,' she wrote back. 'Hormone fluctuations, as every woman knows, can be responsible for breakouts, as can periods of stress. Environmentally, if one is over-using moisturisers or the wrong type of products, or has flown a lot in planes, or has been exposed to lots of environmental irritants and pollutants . . . these are all causes. In addition, some medications aggravate acne, as well as certain internal conditions such as thyroid disease, polycystic ovarian syndrome, or adrenal conditions. Therefore, any sudden onset of acne should be thoroughly investigated by a dermatologist, particularly if it is associated with increased hair growth or loss, which may signal an internal problem that needs addressing.

'The worst case I have ever seen was called *Acne conglobata* and it involved inflamed red pustular bumps and painful nodules all over the face. It was totally disfiguring. We treated it with a combination of steroids (oral and injected), antibiotics and Accutane, and achieved complete clearance. It was very gratifying.'

WINTER SKIN

Having good skin is not just about identifying your skin type, it's about adapting to your skin's different needs, day by day, season by season. In winter moisture evaporates from the skin, caused by central heating and wintry weather. You can do a lot to keep your skin moist before even touching it – put a bowl of water near your radiators to raise the humidity, and avoid sudden dietary changes which will only exacerbate break-outs. Exfoliate the dry-looking skin on the surface, and make sure the moisturiser you use acts as a humectant (bringing water to the surface of the skin), an occlusive (keeping the water in), and an emollient (to smooth and soften the surface of the skin). If your skin is really dry, see a dermatologist, who may prescribe lactic acid in a 12 per cent solution. Do as people in cold countries do: take supplements of cod liver oil to lubricate the skin from within. And make sure you apply your moisturiser well before you go out – unless you want chapped skin – as the cold freezes it.

BAGS UNDER THE EYES

These can sometimes be caused by bad living – over-using cigarettes and alcohol. It doesn't take a dermatologist to tell you, you could just give these up and see an end to the problem. Lack of sleep and sinus problems are also killers for eyes. You can help your skin by brushing it in an upward motion with soft, sable brushes and using an eye mask, or eye gel, both of which should be kept in the fridge. Pat the gel gently around your eyes on the bone, and in this way you will stimulate the circulation as well.

SHADOWS UNDER THE EYES

Dr Polis says that under eye shadows are caused by the following factors:

'Architecture': If the person has protruding lower lid bags, or a deep-set eye, there is a shadow cast below the eye which appears as an under-eye darkness. Only surgical correction will alleviate this.

Heredity: Some peoples, particularly of Indian descent and some Hispanics, have dark areas around the eyes due to their genetic make-up. This is difficult to overcome and we usually end up recommending cosmetic coverage.

Pigmentation: From years of rubbing one's eyes, taking off eye make-up a little too roughly, having allergies, crying now and then, squinting, the delicate tissues of the eye area are prone to having tiny ruptures in the blood vessels, allowing small amounts of invisible blood cells into the surrounding tissues. These blood cells break down and leave brown pigment in their wake. We treat this with eye creams that contain vitamin K to stabilise the blood vessels, and with bleaching ingredients to try and clear the pigment.

Dermatoheliosis: The ageing and sun damage process can leave increased and irregular pigment anywhere on the face, and this area is no exception. We treat this with topical retinoids and topical anti-hydroxy acids, but very slowly and cautiously.

Thinness of the skin: The under-eye area is notoriously thin-skinned, which allows the underlying blood vessels to show through, giving a bluish-brownish hue. We try and plump this skin with the use of non-ablative (or in some cases, ablative) lasers and peels, including Cool Touch lasers, Erbium lasers and CO_2 lasers, and tca peels and phenol peels.

WHOA! WHAT WERE THOSE? – DR POLIS EXPLAINS

Non-ablative lasers: Cool Touch is an example of a non-ablative laser. It stimulates collagen production and decreases the look of wrinkles and scars without removing the top layers of the skin so you can leave the office, have a treatment and go back to work.

Ablative lasers: These include CO_2 and Erbium lasers, which take off the top layers of the skin and you need healing 'down' time.

TCA (Trichloroacetic Acid) peels: These are strong skin peels that will need some down time. They can be given in strengths from 10 per cent to 35 per cent. The stronger the dose, the more down time you'll need, and the better the response.

Phenol peels: There are very strong peels which need to be given by a physician with heart monitoring going on. There is tremendous down time and a high risk of scarring and hyperpigmentation, but when performed correctly they can really rejuvenate a face.

WHAT ANNOYS JACKIE DENHOLM MOORE

Not very much. She is too nice really. And if we do annoy her, she is far too polite to let on. After some persuasion, she eventually tells me, 'The worst thing would be if a client tried to tell you what to do. Another thing is if you've spent ages cleaning the skin, and then they want to put a thick layer of make-up on afterwards. Make sure, when you have a facial, you can just go home and relax. Your hair might look a mess, but it's all about reconditioning the skin. Oh, another thing! People who talk on their mobiles while you're working. That is so irritating. I do understand, they're so busy, but it is difficult.'

SKIN TYPES: DRY/OILY/NORMAL/WHATEVER

How do you know which moisturiser to buy? First by identifying your skin type. This is easier said than done, but Jackie defines skin types and what you should use on them, as follows:

Dry skin is more flaky and parched, with red blotchy marks. It lacks oil and water.

Abject dryness is when it's really flaky and dry. You shouldn't use water at all on the skin. Use a nice, rich, creamy cleansing lotion at night, a gentle toner, and an oil as well as a cream, because an oil is really moisturising and will go deeper into the skin than a cream. In the morning, instead of washing and cleansing the skin again, you should just tone it. Also, regularly exfoliate your skin, because that will free the dead skin, and any cream you use will work more efficiently.

Dehydrated skin feels saggier and looks grey. It doesn't have to be dry. If you pinch it and the pinch mark stays there, then you need to drink more water. Acne skin that gets better is very dehydrated, as is skin that has been subjected to an environmental assault such as sun damage.

Oily skin still needs moisturising. A lot of people with oily skin don't use a moisturiser at all, and their skin just produces more oil because it feels dry. Use a foaming type cleanser with water, trying not to dry out the skin too much. Look for products with antiseptic ingredients, try a stronger toner and products with a mattifying ingredient.

You need to choose products that don't tingle or sting – it might make them feel good in the short term, but that's not helping the skin in the long run. A moisturiser should just feel comfortable on the skin, not tight, or dry. It shouldn't cause break-outs, but leave skin feeling supple.

SKIN TYPES: AN EASY TEST

Cleanse your face and leave it bare for two hours – no moisturiser, no toner, no nothing. Take a sheet of white tissue paper, split it down to its thinnest level, and gently press it over the face. Hold it up to the light. If you have oily skin you'll see patches on the paper; if you have normal or dry skin, the paper will look exactly the same.

How much moisturiser is too much?

'I always say, "Use a Smartie size," says Denholm Moore. Pat it on and then smooth upwards and outwards. If you use too much you will end up massaging more; if you're pulling on the skin then you're not using enough.'

Want to hear a scary story about eye creams?

Save this one for late at night . . . 'I'm a great believer in not overloading the skin,' says Denholm Moore. 'The skin around the eyes is like tissue paper, so if you put too much eye cream on you will overload it. Warm the cream – an amount no bigger than a grain of rice – first in your fingers, then pat it on the bony bit of the eye, very gently. After ten minutes, split a tissue in two and blot the tissue round the area to take off the excess. Most people get puffy eyes because they're putting on too much, too close to the eye.' And the scary bit? 'A plastic surgeon once told me that so many times, he would open up the eye area to do an eyelift, and underneath it would be full of fatty deposits from the overuse of creams. It was completely congested and clogged.'

Is it worth buying anti-ageing creams?

'I don't think anything will get rid of wrinkles once they're there,' says Denholm Moore. 'But prevention is better than cure, so start using an eye cream from 25 plus. Certain eye products will have far more lifting, tightening ingredients in them, whereas with the cheaper makes you will need to put on a lot more product to see any effect, which is counter-productive. All anti-wrinkle products will soften and make wrinkles look better, but no product will take them away permanently.'

Is your new-fangled moisturiser fantastic or a load of old rubbish?

'Get a sample to try first, or put some in a pot so you can go home and try it. Some skins like certain ingredients or textures of creams more than others. Again, you have to go by what your skin is telling you. If your skin is tight, then you're not using a strong enough moisturiser, so change the brand and use something slightly different, or buy an oil or serum to use underneath it. It's very difficult knowing whether it's a load of old rubbish or not. To me, the texture has got to be right. Ask, "I want one that is very light but moisturising" or "I want something thick, but protective." You will know what your skin likes. My skin hates the heavy ones: they cause me to break out. You want a cream that will leave your skin feeling supple and not suddenly bring you out in blackheads. The girl behind the counter should be asking you lots of questions. And you should allow about six weeks of testing before making a decision.'

AND FINALLY: HOW TO HAVE BEAUTIFUL SKIN

Drink lots of water. Get lots of sleep. Try to be happy. Cleanse. Moisturise. And try not to worry too much about getting old. It happens to us all.

'Thirty-five is a very attractive age. London society is full of women of the very highest birth who have, of their own free choice, remained thirty-five for years.'
Oscar Wilde, The Importance of Being Earnest

'I'm thirty-three now, and I don't need to be airbrushed under my eyes.'
Christy Turlington

'All this talk of getting old
It's getting me down my love'
The Verve, 'The Drugs Don't Work'

Chapter Two

MRS COLLAGEN
AND OTHER STORIES

The cops on the corner of Fifth Avenue didn't know when the stationery suppliers they were standing in front of would open. I'd flown in to New York late the night before, only to discover I'd forgotten to pack any tapes for my dictaphone. My day with Dr Laurie Polis, a dermatologist based in SoHo, was all set to start at 9.30, and I didn't want to be late because of a poxy dictaphone tape.

'Let's take a picture anyway!' one of them laughed. They plonked a helmet on my head, thrust a baton in my hand, and there I was, surrounded by four bored policemen, who were gently poking fun at my quaint English ways.

'You're from London. That's in Dublin, right?'

'Er . . . no,' I started, thinking, 'Here we go again, those ignorant Americans,' before they burst out laughing. Even New York cops are wise to that old British bias that assumes all Americans are stupid.

As the shop showed no signs of opening, they put me in a yellow cab and sent me down town. 'There'll be a stationery suppliers there that'll be open by the time you arrive. Don't waste your time waiting for this one. 'Bye now! WE LOVE YOU BRITISH PEOPLE!'

New Yorkers don't like waiting for anyone or anything, but they'll wait for Dr Laurie Polis. Getting appointments with her are like gold-dust – you can wait up to two months. She had offered me a day at her clinic, following her around, watching what she does. Considering there are only 498 consulant dermatologists in Britain (compared with around 10,000 in the USA, according to the American Academy of Dermatology), and that she was at the top of her profession – her client list includes Madonna, Mel Gibson, Drew Barrymore and most of the top models – this was an offer I could not refuse. I arrived at the clinic and introduced myself to one of her assistants, ran out to get the precious tapes, and reappeared, only to wait for what seemed like ages, but was probably only an hour or so in the lobby. Which at least gave me some time to take in my surroundings.

The SoHo Integrated Health Center is no ordinary clinic. For a start, it's unusual to find such a wide range of treatments under one roof. Here you can have everything from lasers, botox and collagen, to peels and microdermabrasion, and the more mundane facials and electrolysis. The environment is also different. In London, if you go and see dermatologists privately, they're usually based in small Harley Street offices. At this clinic, the reception is a vast, loft-style brick and wood affair. There are bamboo poles, coarse grasses and a huge copper circle hanging on the wall. A waterfall runs over frosted glass. Strangely, there are no glossy magazines for patients to read; only leaflets on breast, nose or liposuction surgery. There are lots of copies of *Metro Source New York* – a gay magazine with page after page of advertisements for dermatologists and surgeons. Gay men, it transpires, are under as much, if not more, pressure than women to look good. 'Make the most of every curve,' implore the ads, with lists of things men can do to improve themselves, from fat replacement to penile enhancement and even breast reduction. But there is only one man waiting here, the rest are women – girls who are so tall, slim and pretty it's hard to guess what they're here for.

I read the leaflets about collagen and notice that there is no mention of mad cow disease, which, since collagen is derived from cows, I find rather surprising, but maybe CJD is just a British obsession. The leaflet about botox carries no warnings about pregnancy, which also surprises me – surely if something enters your system, it can also enter your baby's system? And if that thing is a poison? . . .

Botox and collagen, collagen and botox. Isn't it funny how these two little words have slipped so innocently into our beauty consciousness? It is incredible just how much the skincare and cosmetic industry has really changed over the last few years. It used to be there was nothing between moisturisers and facelifts – no intermediary corrective measures, short of the odd acid peel to lift off your skin with all the gusto and gentleness of paint stripper. (One therapist recently told me there is still one peel in use that has pure nail polish remover as its base.) Then skincare companies made several discoveries. Firstly, that Retin-A, a vitamin A topical application formerly used for acne sufferers, could thin the skin and stimulate collagen production – and literally get rid of wrinkles permanently. Secondly, that by injecting collagen – a moisture-retaining protein that comes from animal cartilage – into wrinkles around the mouth area, or into the lips themselves, they could plump up skin that was sagging and bagging and smooth out wrinkles. And finally – perhaps the biggest development of all – they found if they injected a poison, Botulinum Toxin Type A or B – the same strain that causes the disease botulism – into the frown lines by the eyebrows, muscles could be frozen for up to three months at a time, leaving the patient looking much younger, fresher, and certainly less cross. Who needs a facelift any more, if they can have these smaller, less invasive types of on-the-spot surgery? And so the lunch-time lift was born. 'Have your face fixed in your lunch-hour!' screamed the women's magazines. So saturated by this sudden influx of new ways with wrinkles, I had started to believe that at thirty-four, my not having botox or collagen was positively rebellious. Finally! I get to rebel about something.

I wasn't the only one who hated the idea. My cohort, my rebel against the botox bullies, surgery, and pretty much anything unnatural was to be Eve Lom: 'As far as surgery goes,' she said, 'recently I had a woman who had had a facelift done at the age of forty-five. I had not seen her for about six or seven years and she looked a completely different person. She said, "What a shame I had it done, because I will never know how I would have aged." That is enough to put me off and tell women not to get it done. They come to me with three facelifts, and I think, "Why did you bother when you walk like an old woman already?" Lucky, or unlucky, even the best surgeons have their good and bad days. You are at the hands of the knife and that scares me.'

And as for botox itself: 'Everybody is so concerned about eating healthily, fighting pollution . . . You see all these women who have become suffragettes to anti-pollution, anti-deodorants, and yet they turn around the corner and have their faces injected with a poison.'

'That's what I don't understand,' I offer, feebly, unable to compete with her unbridled passion.

'Look, we all have contradictions in ourselves, we are slaves to everything,' she says. 'Botox – these are injections near open sinuses into the forehead, near the eyes and mouth. I don't know, but it scares the hell out of me.'

It scared the hell out of me too, but now it was my turn to find out what it entailed. One of Dr Polis's assistants offered me a white nurse's robe, and suddenly I was on, waiting in a corridor outside four rooms marked Derm 1, Derm 2, Derm 3, Derm 4. So there are four dermatologists, I figured – wrongly, as it turned out. Dr Polis's system, and it's probably a common one, is to line up her patients, get her assistant to interview them, ticking off questions on a long, detailed form, while she flits from room to room.

When Dr Polis arrives, she is a bright ball of energy, with fuchsia pink lipstick and black-rimmed square glasses over dazzling green-blue eyes which are twinkling as she greets me. She assures me it will be fine for me to trail her, tells me I am bound to see some botox, some collagen, maybe a little laser, and that it won't be a problem for her patients to have a journalist 'sit in'. And it isn't a problem. When I explained to one patient who was interested that I was writing a book, she even joked, 'So when I read about the New Mother with Acne, I'll know that's me, right?'

Our first patient is Carrie, and she is so beautiful and with the most perfect coffee-coloured skin that I wonder what on earth she is here for. It transpires she has a fungal rash on her back. It's the kind of thing I could have had for years without even noticing, let alone it bothering me enough to see a dermatologist.

Dr Polis sorts it out: 'It's a yeast infection. It's called *Tinea Versicola* and it comes in many colours. We'll give you something topical for it. You should use a gel for that rash on the elbow, and if that doesn't work, we'll inject it.'

That rash on the elbow looks a little like the one I've had for years and never bothered to do anything about I think to myself.

Carrie has a list of questions ready to ask Dr Polis. She is a regular patient and knows how precious (and how expensive – from $250 for a consultation) time with her derm is. She's not about to waste a minute. 'I was wondering if there was anything I could do about these bags under my eyes.'

You see, that's the thing with being pretty nearly perfect. Any tiny imperfection suddenly takes on an importance all of its own. I swear I couldn't even see these bags, and yet, when they were pointed out to me, . . . well, *was* there anything she could do?

'They could be genetic fat pads. You're young, but this can happen young. You can have surgery for them.'

'How safe is it?' asks Carrie.

'It's always safe in the right hands. The skin lies flat so it doesn't appear puffy any more. You'd have some bruising, and you'd have to wear dark glasses for a while. From a cosmetic point of view in the meantime, use a vitamin C eye cream. You'll feel a difference in a few days.'

Carrie has a tiny, and I mean tiny, scar above her eyebrow and Dr Polis recommends a silicon pad to stick on it to regulate the collagen, which will in turn make it look smoother.

'If that mole on your forehead bothers you, we can remove it.'

Carrie is a model, and that's why she's so thorough at looking after her skin. She gives me a list of shops to visit (hey, I'm in New York), complete with 'Julia Roberts goes there' celebrity descriptions. Suddenly I've lost Dr Laurie. I know she's in Derm 2 but am I allowed in, or not? I knock and enter, to find her removing the stitches from a cyst removal. Yuk. I don't think I need this in my book, so I wait for her to finish and then go with her to her office.

This is clearly where she retreats to between patients, and accounts for why they have to wait so long. This is the hub, her own space, her sanctuary. It's not a very restful sanctuary. For a start there are thirty-seven messages on her answerphone and it's only 11.30 a.m. She has perhaps another sixteen patients to see today, and then, this being Friday, a long drive, weather permitting – to the mountains for some skiing with her children and husband. Her desk is cluttered. The room is small, with none of the bamboo and copper of the reception. But at least there are no patients. Later, back in London, I ask her whether she feels as if she is performing before her patients, as there is an element of the dramatic in her role – the heroine doctor, sweeping in to see a distressed woman, listening to the questions, healing them, giving out the chit-chat, and all in a whistlestop ten minutes. She e-mails me:

> You're right, sometimes interacting with patients (particularly the new ones) is a bit of a performance in the sense that the task is to make an absolute stranger feel comfortable about baring their imperfections, their bodies, and their fears and desires to another stranger, albeit a doctor. I accomplish this often with humour and a sense of ease which patients adopt, and this allows them to relax in an otherwise bizarre and un-comfortable setting. My energy levels remain high because I truly love what I do.

Polis became a dermatologist because she was fascinated by the visual side of it. I had never thought of it as being a particularly visual profession – it's not like she's a painter or film director, for example – but when she explains to me that there are around 4000 known dermatological conditions and even more aspects of cosmetic dermatology all based on visual inspection and the recognition of patterns and morphology, I see what she means. Clearly it's a talent you either have, or you haven't: 'I could see a picture of a skin disease just once in a book, and be able to recognise it even two years later on a living human. I wanted to take advantage of that ability,' she says. I bet she was good at Snap! when she was a kid.

She had bad skin as a teenager and a young adult. 'I used to schlep into this sadistic dermatologist's office every week for his wicked instrument to pick at my pimples and have UV-light treatments. That's a bummer, as I now have to be careful about skin cancers. Finally I had multiple antibiotics and eventually Accutane. Thank God I wasn't a picker and ended up with no scars.'

It was probably this experience that has made her so good with her patients. 'The best I have ever felt after treating a client was after seeing my most severe acne case,' she says. 'A young woman came to see me about a wart on her finger. But when I walked in the room, her face was startling. She had inflamed, pustular, disfiguring extensive acne lesions, virtually covering her face. It was the kind of severe acne (called *Acne Conglobata*) that would have made young children scream and run away. It was shocking. You could barely make out that there was a girl underneath. Yet there she was complaining about a wart on her finger. I quietly discussed her wart, but couldn't resist sensitively bringing up her acne at the end of the visit. I gently suggested to her that she consider allowing me to clear up her skin, which I was confident I could. She burst into tears (she obviously wanted to discuss it, but was so depressed about it that she was avoiding it), and she implored me to try, although others had also tried in the past to no avail. We embarked on an intensive course of topical remedies, antibiotics, surgical injections and treatments. Three months later, she was clear. Clear!! A year later, we lasered away any residual scars, and I can't tell you the change it made in her life. I get teary when I remember this experience.

'Dermatology is fun,' she continues. 'I am able to treat kids, adults and seniors. I am able to prescribe medicine and perform surgery. I can save lives by detecting and treating skin cancer, and I am able to dabble in the less life-threatening aspects such as anti-ageing. I never get bored. I use twelve different lasers, over six different injectibles (collagen, etc.), and am able to radically alter my patients' appearance simply and have a real impact on lives without dealing much with morbidity or mortality.'

I flash her my elbow quickly. 'Is this the same kind of rash that Carrie had?'

'Does it flake?' she asks. 'No? I can get rid of it with a quick injection . . .'

How fantastic. I suddenly realise how inherently British I am after all. It would never occur to me that I could actually get rid of all those niggling annoying little things. I am such a product of the National Health Service that the thought of getting anything minor fixed, privately or otherwise, is a complete anathema.

'That's the best part of being a derm,' says Dr Polis, seeing the delight on my face. 'It's the relationship with the patient. You've got to make a person feel like they're not being judged if they feel concerned about something on their body. If we can get people thinking about their skin, if they come in for a little brown spot they don't like, I might end up finding early melanoma and saving their life.'

Our next patient is a case in point. Angie is here to have her moles checked. Perhaps today was an unusual day but probably every third patient was here to have their moles checked. For a city without much beach, New Yorkers are clearly taking skin cancer very seriously.

'She is blonde, so we're going to keep her safe,' says Dr Polis, injecting a needleful of clear liquid into the base of the mole. The skin puffs up, raising the mole, and with a scalpel, she slices it off, neatly and quickly. The blood rushes to the surface. The detached mole is popped in a bag to be sent off to the lab to find out whether it is cancerous or not. Dr Polis cauterises the skin to stop the bleeding. Eric Clapton is playing in the background. It could have been worse. It could have been that song from *Reservoir Dogs*, where the psycho is slicing his victim to pieces. 'We'll see you in a month,' she says, and my dynamo dermatologist is gone.

When it comes to anti-ageing, what are the concerns of most patients?

Dr Polis: 'I would say that most people, men and women, are concerned about the ageing of their faces in the forties, sometimes in their thirties, but usually their forties. When they're starting to see little lines happening, when they start getting a down-turn in their mouth which reminds them of their grandmother, when they're starting to worry about all the sun they used to have and see discolorations on their face. They come to see me with two qualms: they are concerned about the health of their skin, which is good, and they also want to do something to look a little better, which is healthy psychologically.'

SKINCARE AND SKIN CANCER: WHAT YOU CAN DO TO HELP

Apart from getting your moles checked and wearing sunscreen, you can actually help your skin along by choosing carefully the products that you use.

Dr Polis recommends 'Washing with a glycolic acid cleanser or applying a vitamin C-based moisturiser . . . these are good for both anti-ageing and cancer. Vitamin C helps the skin's immune system resist being suppressed in the state of sunlight. So, although it's not an SPF and it doesn't claim to be an SPF, it will help your skin at another level, fighting the manifestation of skin cancer. Similarly, glycolic acids exfoliate abnormally adherent skin cells by removing the surface dead skin cell layer. Sometimes those early little pre-cancers are just beginning, and they can exfoliate them before they've really taken hold of the skin.

'The only problem is that if you go out in the sun, using vitamin C and glycolic acid can actually leave you more susceptible because they take off the dead skin armour that's sitting on your skin. It's just like having dirt on your skin – we don't consider this as true protection, and yet an adult person who is covered with mud is not going to get burned as easily as a baby who is clean. So it's extra important to protect yourself from the sun when you're using these things.'

What do dermatologists use on their own faces?

Well this one, Dr Laurie Polis, alternates facials with peels and microdermabrasions once a season. 'I use high-quality products at home which have slowly changed from anti-acne to anti-ageing over the years. I currently use a retinoid at night, a vitamin

C in the morning and a glycolic cleanser. I only use moisturiser when necessary – I believe it is greatly overused in America.'

What is a good anti-ageing routine?

Use a sunscreen each morning, and creams containing retinoic acid, vitamin C and occasionally glycolic acid, and you'll be keeping Dr Polis very happy.

MORE SKINOLOGY

Accutane: Accutane is 'isotretinoin' – a synthetic form of high-dose vitamin A often prescribed for acne. It causes many changes in the skin – primarily a closing down of much of the activity of the sebaceous glands, which is the cause of most acne.

Lasers: Lasers are medical devices which do many different things based on the wavelength of the light applied to the skin. For example, for vascular lesions dermatologists choose a wavelength from a laser which is specific for the red in blood vessels so that it selectively destroys those vessels while sparing the rest of the skin.

Microdermabrasion: This is a peel carried out as an in-office procedure where fine crystals or an abrasive device is applied to the skin for short bursts and quickly vacuumed off to 'buff' the skin with no down time. It speeds up the metabolism of the skin, which improves in tone, clarity and texture.

Moles and skin cancer: Aim to get them checked once a year by a qualified dermatologist, but if you have a history of abnormal moles or skin cancer then you should get them checked more frequently.

What is a peel? It's a chemical or physical or mechanical process in which few or many outer layers of the skin are removed for therapeutic purposes.

And now for the real stuff. Our next patient – let's call her Mrs Collagen – is probably in her forties. She is clutching ice to her face, to numb the area that's about to be injected. She has an accent which, with my limited knowledge of New York accents, I would say was more Brooklyn than *Sex and the City*. She is nervous and embarrassed as she has a query about Dr Polis's fees.

'I made a mistake last time. I said I wanted the collagen around my mouth and nose for the same price. I can't spend more than $475.'

Dr Polis is unruffled. It seems like a fair enough comment to me, but later Dr P. tells me she says this every time.

'Okay, well, we'll work to your budget. Do you want the lip lines worked on, or the nasal lines?'

'I think the nasal lines.' Then, to no one in particular, 'I also have to lose at least thirty pounds.'

Dr Polis injects collagen, a milky white liquid, below the small lines. Immediately the lines puff up and flatten into nothing. 'We just raise them up and they're gone,' she says.

Polis works quickly around the mouth and nose area, moving from tiny line to tiny line. 'I knew her skin would take it well. It makes a huge difference. The lines are gone right away. With some patients, if their pores are too big, you shoot the stuff in and it just shoots back. But she's good.'

Amalia, Dr Polis's assistant, wipes the blood away. There isn't much, but it's not an attractive sight, especially as Mrs Collagen still has her lipstick on and it's starting to smudge.

'Does it hurt?' I ask.

'It depends on the patient and their pain tolerance as to how much injections hurt. But they're all tested for allergic reactions to collagen beforehand,' says Dr Polis.

Suddenly Mrs Collagen says, 'I thought that side was worse,' and moves her arm upwards to point to the wrinkles, jogging Dr Polis in the process.

'Hey! I have a needle in my hand!' says Dr Polis, rather more calmly than I probably would have in the circumstances.

She apologises yet again. Dr P. keeps going.

'You know, the biggest complaint I have about collagen is that it doesn't last – about six months in the face,' says Dr Polis. 'Restylane lasts twice as long, but we can't get it here, it hasn't been FDA approved yet.'

'But everyone's different, and it lasts longer in some patients than others. If you go eating steak or apples just after you've had it done, it won't last so long. Now . . .' she says to Mrs Collagen, 'Now, this is a whole syringe, but we've only used two-thirds, so we'll save the rest for another time, and that way we'll be sticking to your budget. Don't talk too much for two to three hours afterwards, and if anyone asks why you can't talk, just say you've been to the dentist.'

As soon as Dr Polis leaves the room, Mrs Collagen starts complaining to Amalia. 'Did she remove the bigger lines? I don't think she removed the bigger lines. Did she get rid of them? I really don't think she removed the bigger lines. Can you see?' she asks, anxiously.

Mrs Collagen's skin is looking smoother, better, and, it's true, there are still a few lines left, but overall there is definitely an improvement.

'She did the best she could but she was trying to respect your budget,' says Amalia, incredibly patiently. 'She got all the others. It looks fine.'

'But I wanted to wear my hair back!' she complains.

This is what I would have said if I was Amalia: 'Look. Your hair is back already and your lines are next to your mouth. The lines are not going to make the slightest bit of difference to whether you wear your hair back or not. Your face is orange because you are wearing the wrong foundation for your skin colour. Sorting that out alone would knock ten years off you.'

Later, I see how collagen is used not just to puff up and get rid of wrinkles temporarily, but how it can work to great effect on skin that is bumpy, or just a bit craggy. And not all of Dr Polis's collagen patients are as annoying as Mrs Collagen.

When is your skin suitable for collagen?

When you're noticing wrinkles and/or lines caused by excessive squinting, frowning, smoking and smiling. If you have scars, collagen can pad them out and make the skin appear smooth. Fewer than 1 per cent of patients can be allergic to bovine collagen but you should still have a sample skin test before your treatment.

What is Restylane?

'It's a new injectable for the correction of wrinkles and scars which is comprised of a natural sugar substance found in the skin,' says Dr Polis. 'It has no protein in it and does not require a skin test. It lasts longer than traditional collagen but hurts more going in. It has not yet been approved for use in the USA, but is used in Canada, Europe and Asia.'

What areas respond best to collagen replacement treatments?

This is one of the questions that appears in the collagen leaflet at Dr Polis's clinic. 'The ten areas most frequently treated with collagen are: frown lines between the eyes, acne scars, cheek depressions, smoker's lines around the mouth, marionette lines at the end of the mouth, worry lines in the forehead, crow's feet at the eyes, deep smile lines, dimples and facial scars.' (And, by the way, she's not talking about cute dimples, à la Kirk Douglas.)

How many treatments are necessary?

A typical patient has bigger 'defects' treated in two or three treatments over a three-month period, with maintenance after that depending on how long it lasts (from two to six months).

How effective is collagen in anti-ageing creams?

'We have known since the 1970s that topical collagen does nothing. It must be injected for it to effect a change. Having collagen in skincare topical products is like selling snake oil,' says Dr Polis. At best, collagen in moisturisers is a good humectant, and these days it is more likely to be derived from plants or marine sources.

However, don't dismiss some of the collagen-producing ingredients such as topical vitamin C, and topical retinoids in skincare – these do help boost the skin's production of collagen.

Skincare companies like Estée Lauder stopped using animal-derived collagen in their skincare products years ago, and obviously in Britain, we're not so keen on the idea of injecting bovine-derived collagen into our faces. Is it safe to use collagen like this?

Dr Polis says, 'Yes, because the cows used for injectable collagen are sequestered and do not have disease.'

What happens to the collagen after it is injected into the skin?

It is slowly metabolised over the next two to six months.

One thing I often hear from Dr Polis is how she enjoys the dual aspects of her work: doing the 'fun' anti-ageing stuff as well as the 'more serious stuff'. It's not just cancers. It's the woman who comes to see her with a terrible case of rosacea – 'It's not going to kill you, but the bad news is it's not curable, only controllable' – to whom she administers a rosacea cream made by a fellow-dermatologist, and cautions to use vegetable-based cleansers and sunscreen and to avoid steam rooms, spicy foods and red wine. Another patient is having laser treatment to remove small bumps on the skin caused by the sebaceous glands growing too much (*Sebaceous hyperplasia*). They could be treated with a topical antibiotic, but they would only grow back. Lasering removes them permanently. As we stand over her, in plastic goggles to protect our eyes, she cautions her patient that 'this may hurt'.

'Take a deep breath, the first few hits are a little uncomfortable. Here's a beauty. How're you doing under there? Look at that, do you see it vaporising away. See all of those big bumps? See how we just got rid of them? Sorry about leaning on you, are you okay? Anything I do that makes you uncomfortable you just speak up, baby, okay?'

She is constantly referring to a scrappy diagram she has drawn, marking roughly where the bumps are. It's not meant to be precise – precision comes from what she actually sees as she leans over the patient, but at least it guides her as to where to look. The laser makes a short, sharp tapping sound. Her patient doesn't complain.

'You will look like someone with chicken pox for a couple of days.'

The patient who I feel most sorry for, is an older lady – not that sixty or so is at all old these days. She has had unusual 'dermal lesions which might be an auto-immune response'. In other words, her rash might indicate the presence of something horrible going on inside. Somehow I am left sitting in Derm 1 with her for a good half-hour while Amalia and Dr Polis search for the results of her biopsy. She is quiet, obviously very intelligent, a chic New Yorker, with silver-grey hair. Yet she sits there, waiting patiently, in a pair of big knickers and a T-shirt, covered with a paper towel.

I offer her some water to drink. I make small talk. I want her to ask me about me, not in some 'me, myself, I' kind of way, but because I don't want to have to ask her about herself. Suddenly every topic of conversation is too personal. I can't ask about September 11th (this is only a few months later), because she probably knows someone who died, and I don't want her to feel distressed. I obviously can't ask her about her skin, which is red and inflamed from the rash. I make my excuses and leave her to wait with Eric Clapton. She probably looked nervous and uncomfortable because I was bugging the hell out of her anyway.

Back to the fun stuff, as Dr Polis would say – namely: botox. Perhaps it was just that day, but her botox clients seemed to be the most sophisticated of all. There was the Waspy-type girl with a huge diamond ring on her engagement finger and a black Barbour jacket. Then there was the art dealer ('Jay [Jopling] is kind of a friend of mine'), who was off the next day to London for gallery auctions and wanted a little 'fix' in time for her trip. Disappointingly, there is not much to write about. The devil doesn't jump out from nowhere and tell you you've sold your soul to Vanity. There is no picture of Dorian Gray up in the attic. The patients don't break out into pustulent rashes or fall into uncontrollable muscle spasms. Instead, they chat calmly away to Dr Polis while she injects their faces with a clear liquid.

'Let me see your crows,' she begins, referring to the crow's feet around their eyes. The patient signs a consent form.

'Okay, now look straight at my nose. Really push your eyebrows together and then release.'

The skin bumps up where the botox goes in.

'Botox is quick, easy, there's no down time,' says Dr Polis. 'There is no other procedure that can do what botox comes up with.' Like anything, however, it only works when it's in the right hands. Too many injections in the wrong place can freeze the muscles in the wrong position, or cause an eyebrow to droop. 'The tricky thing about the eye area is that there are small veins, and if you get near them you can bruise.'

My WASP bride-to-be sits there holding gauze pads over the mosquito bite-sized bumps that have sprung up on her forehead, to absorb the small dots of blood that appeared when the needle went in. She is fine, she looks happy. In a matter of three days her wrinkles will be gone. And now so will Dr Polis, this time for the weekend. It's 4 p.m., it's Friday, and seventeen patients later, her day is over.

BOTOX

HOW DOES IT WORK?

Botox blocks the impulses that run from the nerve to the tiny facial muscles which move when we express ourselves. This relaxes the muscles so they do not contract. In practice, this means that the skin in the treated area looks smooth and unwrinkled, while the rest of the face moves in a normal expression. You won't be able to scowl, but you can laugh. Perfect for those passive-aggressive types.

ARE YOU READY FOR IT?

Yes, if worry lines, frown lines, laughter lines, crow's feet and other dynamic wrinkles are looking a little too permanent. Yes, if it doesn't bother you that you can't look really cross when you're having an argument. Yes, if you can afford it – it's not cheap, and when you've had it once (and if you're happy with the results) you'll need to have injections about two to three times a year to maintain the look.

No, if the wrinkles that bother you are caused by general ageing and sun-damaged skin, since these are unrelated to facial muscle contractions. No, if you are over sixty-five years of age – the duration of effect (usually from three to six months) varies from patient to patient, but is less effective over sixty.

And now for those questions for The Expert. . .

Is it safe to inject a poison into your skin?
'Well, it's true,' says Dr Polis. 'In its unrefined, undiluted, unsterilised, undesiccated and unreconstituted form, and at 64,000 times the dose we inject, botox IS a poison. But remember that penicillin comes from a fungus . . . ugh! Who would want to ingest a fungus? We don't even think of it that way, though we realise its medical benefit. There are basically no side effects to Botox except that if the person lies down immediately after the injection, it may diffuse into unwanted areas and cause eyelid drooping, which is subtle and temporary, but is rare. Exceedingly rare complaints may include transient double vision or headaches. But botox is a perfect treatment as far as I'm concerned. It has little or no risks, does without surgery what nothing else can do, takes a short time, and effects positive changes.'

What happens to the botox once it's been put into the skin?
It is taken up by the neuromuscular junction anatomy and is slowly metabolised over the next four to eight months.

Is it advisable to have it while pregnant?

'Botox does not travel through the bloodstream, it does not cross the placenta, nor is it excreted in breast milk. It is safe!' says Dr Polis.

Not everyone agrees. Some dermatologists I spoke to would be unwilling to take such responsibility. Perhaps this uncertainty exists because botox has only really been around for seven years or so and we simply can't be sure. Perhaps it's because, with so many new botox operators around with much less experience, there is more chance of a mistake. Personally, I wouldn't take the risk. No wrinkle is worth it.

Of course, the final frontier in getting your face fixed is literally just that – getting your face fixed. With big knives. No, not really, they're probably skinny scalpels, but you can't help but be a little dramatic when it comes to talking about surgery. We've all seen the horror stories, the TV programmes where surgeons left perfectly beautiful faces scarred for life; where patients have been left to recover in almost squalid conditions because they flew out to some second rate doctor's office in an obscure part of Eastern Europe – all in a bid to cut costs.

Because there is so much about surgery that can go wrong, it's a blessing that there are women like Wendy Lewis around. Lewis spent twelve years working in plastic surgeons' offices in New York counselling patients and assistant surgeons and then decided, *Enough already*! Why not set up her own business doing it? She now matches her clients with the right surgeon, dental technician, or even facialist for them. Her business has been so phenomenally successful – she is completely independent so her clients know they are getting an unbiased opinion and not just some 'You scratch my back, I'll scratch yours' referral – that, as with Dr Polis, you can expect to wait months for an appointment with her. Best of all, she has a lovely bedside manner – you would want to tell this woman all your problems, not just those relating to your looks. Based in New York, when she visits London it is not uncommon for her to have eight one-hour in-person consultations back to back, starting at 8 or 9 a.m. and going straight through the day. Who are her clients?

'A typical day might start with a GP from Manchester who is curious about botox, then a bank secretary from London who wants breast implants, next a solicitor from Leeds interested in a facelift, followed by a mother of three from Birmingham who needs a tummy tuck, and a make-up artist from Essex who is thinking about having the bump on her nose removed,' she says. Each of her clients has their own set of demands and requirements, all of which need to be translated according to their priorities and budgets. Invariably, her appointments run over time, as patient after patient gets talking not just about their physical dreams, but sometimes their emotional triggers. 'I often tell them not to have surgery at all – for example, if I think the surgery is not safe or effective, or that I don't think it will make them happy.'

Lewis is a firm believer in skincare first – not over-moisturising, but concentrating on cleansing, exfoliating and sun protection – and then not smoking, and drinking only in moderation. 'Sun, smoke and drink age people most rapidly and are all within your control. No excuses,' she says. 'Add to that keeping your weight stable, and you're doing the best you can. A great hairstyle and make-up means you're more than halfway there. And wearing a smile never hurt either – happy women are pretty women, they exude confidence and sexiness.'

The question is: how do you know that you're in the right hands? Ultimately, it's your decision, and for that, you have to do the research. This is one instance when listening to your best friend is not enough. Forget about small ads in newspapers and magazines – they're just too dicey as you don't know what you're getting. This is a surgeon you're trying to find, not a villa in Tuscany or a good florist or caterer.

'If they have to advertise, it's never a good sign,' says Lewis. 'Anyone can post anything on the Internet without being subject to substantiation. Besides, what really counts is not the clinic, but the surgeon within the clinic, as well as the quality of the anaesthetist.' She advises being wary of doctors who present a prepared list of references, heavily commercialised websites, brochures, videos and ads that promise big discounts or look just a little too slick.

Instead, you should be requesting brochures and developing a list of questions ready to ask at a consultation. Make sure the surgeon is a reputable member of an organisation of surgeons who specialise, and that he has a documented education, has completed a formal training programme and has extensive experience in performing the procedures you are considering. (You'd be surprised.)

'The real gift in cosmetic surgery is as much in the eyes as it is in the hands,' says Lewis. 'If you know what beauty is but can't deliver it, it's just as tragic as knowing how to operate but being devoid of a sense of aesthetics.' When Wendy Lewis looks for a surgeon, she is just as interested in his sense of creativity, raw talent and innovation as she is in his diplomas. It is vital that he also has an interest in learning new techniques, while still caring about his patients and having a good rapport with them. 'You don't have to fall in love with your surgeon, but you should at least like and respect him. If you are afraid or intimidated by your cosmetic surgeon, you will be too timid to ask the right questions and get the answers you need. It also helps if he likes you. If he can't stand the sight of you, you won't get his best work, period. So don't go antagonising him: keep your appointments, pay your bills on time, and thank him when you are happy. It means more than you can imagine.'

For most women embarking on surgery, the first surgical procedure they opt for is, according to Lewis, an 'eyelid rejuvenation'. This involves removing the eye bags from the lower lids, or removing a strip of skin from the upper lid crease, or both. 'Having a little conservative work done around the eyes can make a world of difference to the way you look and feel. When you look tired, even when you are in fact well-rested, it usually means your eyes are showing some wear and tear.'

If your surgeon is a good one, he will look at your face and see instantly what needs improvement, but he will also evaluate you as an individual. Character in a face is a good thing. 'Not every woman should have a nose without a bump,' Lewis says. 'On some faces, it would look silly. Cosmetic surgery should never be undertaken to please someone else, or just because the surgeon thinks it should be done. Just because he can make it better, doesn't mean to say he should.'

A small amount of surgery can sometimes make a big difference. 'One thing that makes a major change to your look is a chin implant if you have a weak bone structure,' says Lewis. 'It changes the entire shape of the face and creates facial harmony. Brilliant improvements can be had with a little piece of silicone rubber. A subtle rhinoplasty – making a big nose smaller, or reducing a bump – can also make all the difference between ugly duckling and beauty. But less is always more,' she cautions. 'One well-done, careful facelift will not make you look like a freak. Becoming unrecognisable is usually the result of multiple, aggressive procedures via surgery, injections, implants to the skin itself, performed frequently over a long period of time, and often by several surgeons in numerous continents. The skin is a living organ that can withstand only so much assault before it begins to take on an unnaturally shiny or waxy appearance.'

Your state of mind has to be rock-solid as well. Not only do you have to know when you're being pressurised into having more surgery than you really want to – Lewis tells of one doctor who even tells prospective patients he will make them look like Catherine Zeta-Jones or Brad Pitt – but if you are clinically depressed, have 'low self-esteem issues', are in an abusive relationship, are grossly overweight, or in poor health, you should not even be considering it. 'If you are mentally, or emotionally unstable, it is a recipe for disaster,' says Lewis. 'Surgery rarely changes your life in the way you might expect it to; it doesn't make your husband suddenly rekindle his undying passion for you, or get you a great job or a new home, or a spot on network television, or a part in De Niro's next movie.'

Another major reason why some people are not good candidates is that they have totally unrealistic expectations about what can and cannot be accomplished from surgery. Doctors aren't miracle-workers. Worse still – and we've all seen pictures of Jocelyne Wilderstein – is the danger that you could become addicted. It can have a similar effect to mood-enhancing drugs, but this time you are in serious danger of becoming a 'cosmetic surgery junkie'. 'Women go to great lengths to achieve physical perfection. Cosmetic surgery should not be looked upon as a fashion statement, fad or craze.'

Surgery, as I said before, really is the last resort. In 1991, Naomi Wolf wrote in her book on beauty and the ideology of women, *The Beauty Myth*: 'We have entered a terrifying new age with cosmetic surgery. All limits have broken down. No amount of suffering or threat of disfigurement can serve as a deterrent. What is happening to the female body in relation to cosmetic surgery is like what is happening to the balance of life on the planet. We are at an historic turning point.'

I hate to say it, because I refuse to be judgemental about cosmetic surgery, botox, collagen and the rest, and those who opt for it, but I do sometimes wonder if she is right. It does seem as if no amount of pain is too much; as if no little flaw is too small; no price too much to pay in the pursuit of beauty. I know that I am a part of that industry, and that writing about it can make what used to be extra-ordinary, ordinary, but it doesn't mean that I am totally at ease with this side of it. If it makes you happy, go and do it, is what I say – just do it with someone you trust. But if somewhere along the line you can consider whether it is really the way you look that makes you unhappy, as opposed to your miserable job, your weight, your health, your husband, your childhood . . . then put it off. God made us the way we are, after all.

Look, ask me again in ten years, when gravity has really taken its toll.

WHAT QUESTIONS SHOULD YOU ASK YOUR SURGEON?

Wendy suggests the following:

Does the doctor have hospital privileges and where?
Your surgeon should maintain an association with at least one or several fully licensed hospitals or clinics.

Is the doctor's surgery facility accredited and how long has it been in business?
Freestanding hospitals and clinics require regulation and are subject to frequent inspection according to national, regional and local standards.

What are the risks and complications of the procedure?
A reputable doctor will start with the 'D' word (DEATH) and work his way down to infection and bad scars. Never tell the doctor that you don't want to know; it is as much your responsibility to find out as it is his responsibility to inform you.

How long will the procedure take?
Surgeons have a natural tendency to downplay the extent of the surgery. They are not always being deliberately misleading: they are just being 'surgeons'. If your surgeon says the procedure will take six or more hours, get a second opinion to see if that amount of time is reasonable for the operation proposed.

How long will the results last?
This translates into 'When will I need to do it again?'

How long will I take to heal?
This question is impossible to answer with any degree of certainty. No surgeon can promise you that you'll be bruise-free by any given date.

How much time will I have to be out of work? Or when can I fly home? Or when can I drive?

Ask about anything that applies to your lifestyle to aid you in planning your time and recruiting help to drive you to and from the doctor's rooms for suture removals and check-ups.

What type of anaesthesia will be given and who will be administering it?

Anaesthesiologists are medically trained specialists that first have to become medical doctors and then complete a residency. The options of local or general anaesthesia are discussed with both the anaesthesiologist and your surgeon.

If I don't like the result, what can be done?

Surgery is not a perfect science, so make sure your doctor stands behind his work and is willing to do what it takes to make you happy (within reason, of course).

What are the alternatives?

If you decide not to have the surgery the doctor is recommending, find out what else you can do to improve the feature you are complaining about or to make yourself look prettier, softer, younger, etc . . .

If I were your sister/daughter/wife, would you tell me to have the surgery?

Look him straight in the eyes when you ask this. It's harder to give a trumped-up answer to a direct question like this, but save it for last.

ARE YOU REALLY READY FOR PLASTIC SURGERY?

- You must be in good health, and any procedure you consider should be safe and effective with limited risks that are acceptable to you. NEVER take unnecessary risks.
- You should be able to afford to have something done without it being a

financial hardship. In such cases, far too much will be riding on the outcome of surgery.

- Do your homework, and always ask a lot of questions.
- NEVER go with the first surgeon or doctor you consult. Always see at least one more. Get a second opinion for everything.

WHAT ANNOYS WENDY LEWIS

'I can't stand faces and anatomy that have been distorted – pulled too tight, scars that are visible, obvious tell-tale signs of cosmetic alterations. These are not examples of good work. Good surgery should be undetectable – fine, clean scars placed correctly, elegantly executed surgeries, these are the most important aspect of it all. For me, badly done surgery is the worst sin. Noses that are too small or too short, tight eyelids, over-lifted brows, all these things make you look older than your chronological age.'

LEWIS'S ALL-TIME FAVOURITE BEAUTY TIP

This has nothing to do with surgery. 'Wear make-up – it covers a multitude of sins. All the cosmetic surgery in the world won't do what wearing concealer, lipstick, foundation and mascara can do for you. I find it a big challenge to get women to wear enough make-up to really enhance their looks, including myself. I have learned from make-up artists that the older you get, the more definition you need in your face.'

DIY PLASTIC SURGERY – HERE'S ONE YOU CAN TRY AT HOME . . .

Hamilton is a hairstylist and make-up artist who often works on the sets of pop promos and celebrity shoots. These scalpel-free suggestions are things he has done time and time again to performers – for film premieres, videos and other occasions.

HAMILTON'S FACELIFT

'Taping the face is a real skill. It's very effective if you get it right and will take at least ten years off you.' The best tapes are those which you can buy from a good make-up suppliers, such as ScreenFace. It's stronger than medical tape. Start by lifting the eyes. On clean, i.e. make-up-free skin, apply the tape near the temple but close to the hairline using the hook to fix a piece of string or elastic on to the tape near the temple. Pull the string over the head, through the hair and up around the back, to the other temple, then hook the thread on to the other tape. You can lift the eyes as much as you want – it works exactly the same way as a facelift, in that you are moving the folds of skin up into the hairline. Use the hair at the front of the head to hide the tapes at the temples. Then lift the jaw in exactly the same way – tape under the jawline and then up, under and round the head to pull the skin up from the neck area. Hide the tapes with hair by the ear-lobes.

HAMILTON'S BOOB JOB

Medical tape is best for this, but if you're stuck, you can use gaffer tape. Push your breasts together to see how you would like them to look. Try on your dress or corset, or whatever outfit you will be wearing, and adjust your breasts to form the shape you want. If necessary, mark with an eyeliner (pick a shade slightly darker or lighter than your skin colour which will be easier to remove afterwards). Remove your outfit. Take the tape and run it around the back and over the breasts, as if you are creating a bra with it. You can create a cup under the armpits as far as it will show. Afterwards, wipe off the markings, and remove the pencil-marks.

'There is no easy way to get the tape off afterwards, it's a no-pain, no-gain story,' Hamilton says.

It's still a whole lot less painful than surgery (although the results obviously won't last so long).

HAMILTON'S INSTANT TUMMY TUCK

'This is great for wearing under a slip dress for an event where you have to turn up and sit down – although you might not feel like eating much.

'Take a roll of cling film and stick a long strip of medical tape along one length, holding the tube vertically. Stick the cling film to your spine, then wrap the film round and round to create a flexible corset.'

HOW DO MODELS IN MAGAZINES GET SUCH PERFECT SKIN? ASK THE ART DIRECTOR.

The art director is one of the most important people on a magazine's staff – second only to the editor, and on some magazines, actually on a par with the editor. Art directors set the style for the magazine, supervising the photographic shoots, the graphics and other images that make up that magazine.

'I like the fact that as an art director, the world arrives on your desk,' says British *Vogue*'s Robin Derrick, who is also a photographer and arguably one of the best art directors in the business. He works only two floors upstairs from me at *Tatler*, but he's so busy I had to practically stalk him for this interview every time he passed my office on the way to Tony's coffee shop. When I finally track him down he shows me a picture he has taken himself, and then worked on with his computer. The model has skin that looks so creamy soft you could almost reach into the picture and touch it. Her skin was pretty near perfect to begin with, but by digitally manipulating the picture he has managed to give a depth to both eyes, including the one that is further away that would normally have been out of focus, as well as remove any tiny blemishes. He can clone whole areas of skin, and move them to cover other areas of the face – a bit like a surgeon's cutting and pasting. The picture is astonishingly real, life-like and three-dimensional as a result, and yet it's still a picture, it's still distant.

Is retouching the ultimate plastic surgery?

*Derrick says: 'I take pictures that are warts and all, and then I work on them after-
wards – that's not the way most photographers work, but it is the way I work. I think
that in photography, the first base of retouching is that no one wants a permanent
reminder of a temporary blemish. Retouching at this level is totally acceptable. But
I do think that digital processing has become a little over-used, with a whole genre
of photography springing up where girls look like shop mannequins, which is all to
do with 3-D, virtual reality, Gameboy things. At one end of the scale you have this
brilliant quote from the photographer Nick Knight, "Digital technology has released
photography from its duty to be truthful" so that "the camera never lies" will never
be a true expression again. And yes, we are in the realms of image-making, so the
notion that there is a nobler picture is spurious, as every picture has an angle, a light,
and is a part of the craft of photography. It's a bit like synchronised music – it's
fabulous, just as an acoustic guitar is brilliant. You do see a lot of retouching in
beauty advertising, partly because it goes through so many committee decisions with
everyone getting involved. But the over-airbrushed stuff will pass, I hope.'*

*By the way, in case you're wondering, the man whose task it is to make women
look as glorious, glamorous and sexy as only* Vogue *models can, is himself a rather
burly, almost scruffy kind of guy. But very nice.*

'If all the girls in this beauty contest were laid end to end, no one would be the least bit surprised.'
Dorothy Parker

Chapter Three

'DIDN'T YOU USED TO BE A MODEL?'

Maida Vale, London W9. I lived in Maida Vale once, in a small but perfectly formed flat on the top floor of a block of four. I had a horrible freeholder who charged a fortune in service charges for services we never had. There was a wonderful little Greek restaurant around the corner, where two ladies, as wide as they were tall (and they weren't that tall), would serve retsina and kleftiko. There was a tennis court off Elgin Avenue with a secret indoor bowling green with painted murals around the sides. And there was the Glauca Rossi make-up school, which I must have walked past a thousand times, each time wondering: Was it any good? Who went there? And was Glauca that funny Italian woman who'd done my make-up once some five years or so ago?

It's now ten years ago, and yes, she was that woman, and yes, the school is good, if one is to go by the success of some of her former pupils. In that funny way fate has of presenting you with a collection of little coincidences all at once, compelling you to put two and two together and act on your instincts, I decided to go to Glauca's school and see for myself. A press release – not particularly well written – arrived on my desk one day, about the school the Italian make-up artist runs for would-be professionals. That same week, I had worked with another make-up artist called Melanie Arter, who did the most beautiful make-up on the model Catherine Hurley for a *Tatler* feature, and who told me she'd trained at Glauca's school. And then I discovered that Charlotte Tilbury, who is one of today's make-up 'stars' (anything to avoid that over-used expression, 'make-up artist of the moment') and is a friend, also trained there. I booked myself in.

The PR seemed a little suspicious at first. Why would I want to attend the course? It was intended for professionals and ran over twelve weeks, so I might not find it very exciting. Could I come for just an afternoon? Then I could see a demonstration on models. No, I wanted a day, at least, and I wanted to be treated just like a student. I wanted to be applying make-up, just like a student – in fact that was the whole point. I was advised to bring a notebook.

I love writing about make-up. Going backstage at the shows to report on the goings-on of make-up artists and hairstylists is about as close to being a 'real' journalist as a beauty editor can get. The atmosphere backstage is electric, even when it's relatively quiet and boring and everyone is hanging around gulping down mineral water and puffing on cigarettes. Identifying a Val Garland, or a Stephane Marais, or a Pat McGrath, watching from afar, and then inching as close as possible without annoying them, asking questions, taking notes, observing . . . give me this over a skincare launch any day. Which is why I have never understood why people (by people, I really mean editors, and my sister Fiona) dismiss the shows as being 'irrelevant'. 'They're the lifeblood!' I argue. 'Oh, come *on*. Who wears that kind of make-up anyway?' they retort, by which they usually mean the one show they've seen where the make-up artist – okay, I admit it – went a little too pantomime with the blue eyeshadow.

I'll tell you who wears that kind of make-up. Ordinary women. Take a look around the next time you get on a bus, order dinner in a restaurant, or go to the theatre, and you'll see that the person sitting next to you is also a fan of the blue eyeshadow. Sometimes it's tastefully done, sometimes it isn't, but I'm convinced that deep down we're all make-up enthusiasts at heart.

But as much as I love writing about make-up, I have a pathological fear of it. I never wear any, beyond concealer, mascara, blush, and lip gloss. I can't do it. I have neither the patience nor the skill, and I don't want to spend months practising how to do a straight black line on my upper lids, thank you very much. I just want to pop it on, then take it off when it's all over. Also, and I suspect I'm not the only one here, I feel guilty thinking about it at all. A strange perception for someone whose job it is to write about it, perhaps, but there is something about make-up that implies sheer vanity in a way that doesn't apply to the way we think about skin- or haircare, which are somehow more about maintenance.

All of which pointed strongly to my doing the course. How could I write about applying make-up if I couldn't put the stuff on myself? I decided to do some research first, so I called Barbara Daly. Daly has been a make-up artist for about a thousand years, but became really famous when she did Lady Diana Spencer's make-up for her ill-fated wedding to Prince Charles. I suppose you could say that Diana was her most famous make-up 'pupil'. What was she like?

'I remember the day I met her,' says Daly. 'We were a very similar build and the same height, and she said, "It's not often I can look another woman straight in the eye." Daly continued to work for her for years after that, and the pair kept in touch, with the always impeccably turned out Diana becoming very good at doing her own make-up, thanks mainly to two things. 'She had the benefit of experts,' says Daly, 'but she was also very interested herself. She'd find out how to take that expertise and adapt it to suit her, and learn how to do things. She would actually listen. You can give someone a lesson on how to do their make-up, and they will love it, but they won't practise themselves.'

Daly's own teaching method for one-to-one lessons involves making up half a client's face, then getting the client to do the other half herself. Apparently, one of the hardest things about teaching is getting a person to learn how to look. 'You have to learn how to use your eyes. You have to see the details,' she says. Then there are the other skills that professionals have learnt, like finding the right light to sit in, holding a brush or a sponge the correct way, and acquiring the right techniques. 'There is a lot of emphasis on make-up, on colours, but you can have drawers full of cosmetics that you don't know what to do with, and it's such a waste.'

The other important thing, Daly says, is: 'Be realistic. Fine eyeliners, how dexterous are you really? Someone might come to me and say, "I couldn't paint a line on my eyes because my hand shakes." "Well," I say to them, "what is it you like about the look? Let's take that aspect and see what you can do." The same goes for the time element. You have to make the best of your time, if you only have ten minutes in the morning. You also need to learn how to edit. If you have terrific skin, what is the point in wearing foundation every day just because it's a given rule? Learn what works for you. That, actually, is what experts have to offer.'

I will look and I will listen. I will acquire a technique. I will acquire several techniques. I will make the best of my time. I will learn how to edit. I will learn what works best for me. These are my mantras when I finally arrive at Rossi's school.

I ring the wrong doorbell. There are three or four Japanese students standing outside, and a couple of Englishy-looking ones, but I only notice the Japanese because, as usual, they are looking super-fashionable in a weird *iD* magazine kind of way that only Japanese students can. 'Try the top bell if you want Glauca,' says one of the Englishy-looking ones, smiling. I am obviously not about to be treated like a normal student, but it's a bit hopeless expecting to work 'under cover' when I'm dropping in for one day only and the others have all been here for eight weeks already.

Rossi sits upstairs in a bright, if a little shabby, room, with her back to the street and a signed Norman Parkinson photograph on the wall behind her. The sun is streaming in. I don't know if she smokes, as she has a bad cold today, but she must have done at some point to have earned such a fantastically gravelly voice. She is friendly, intriguing – a woman with lots of stories to tell in her rich Italian accent. In her own way she is a little nervous of me, although probably not as nervous of me as I am of her and her class, which, as Melanie has told me, is difficult, intense, and Rossi herself is not without her moments. She moved from Milan to London in the 1970s and worked with Norman Parkinson and Bruce Weber for *Vogue*, before opening her school in 1989. She has that natural teacher's authority. She is also checking me out.

'Have we met before?' she asks.

'I don't think so. I'm not sure.'

'Did you used to model?' she says.

'Yes. Maybe I met you then,' I reply. I am deliberately being evasive because I remember having my picture taken for some test shots for which Rossi had done the make-up. They were nice enough, as I remember, but I don't want our past encounter, although more than amicable – to colour today's work. It's embarrassing. It wouldn't be so bad if I had been a half-decent model, but I wasn't. I was always the short fat one on the end. Quite literally in one instance, when in one of the more credible things I ever did – a Bella Freud show video filmed by Kate Garner – there was Susie Bick and ten other pretty, young things, and there was I, the short fat thing on the end. I was mostly edited out. 'Never mind, you'll get bread and butter work,' said my agency. And I did, a whole loaf-full of it, from *Bella* covers to Marks and Spencer's bra packets. They're in storage somewhere, waiting for the day they will miraculously metamorphose from naff to kitsch. Which is why I don't want my cover to be blown.

We pass downstairs to a large room equipped with mirrors, bright lighting and professional-looking trays of colours, brushes and sponges in an ordered chaos in front of each student. A sign on the wall lists the rules and regulations: no chewing gum; no food; and no drinks (other than water). I am introduced and offered as a model to Julie, who will make me up first before we swap around, and I get to make her up. Although everyone is concentrating hard, the atmosphere is relaxed. Rossi walks around, checking on her students' work as they apply foundation. 'Julie,' she says, as Julie gets to work on my spots and bags. 'Use a pink and yellow tinted concealer under the eyes: it counteracts any grey or green in under-eye circles. On a spot you would use a pure yellow tinted concealer as you don't want to accentuate any redness.' (Thanks for pointing them out to everyone, Glauca.)

When everyone has applied foundation, the twelve of us assemble around Rossi for a demonstration of a 'fashion look'. It's essentially a monochrome look on matt skin, with heavy brown eyes finished with a touch of black eyeliner, shading under the cheekbones, and pale lips to contrast with the eyes. 'Everything goes round in circles,' says Rossi. 'I used to do this shading under the cheeks in the Eighties.'

It looks simple, and everyone is enthusiastic and sets to work straight away. By the time we swap round and I am making up Julie, I have rehearsed how I am going to recreate the look in my head so many times, I am sure it will only take me a few minutes. But it's not that easy. Where do I put my hands? Am I allowed to put one on Julie's head to help me steady my other hand? Or on her chin when I am doing her lips? And am I dragging her skin? Did I just poke her in the eye? Maybe she's just being polite? About halfway through doing the eyes I realise I am now pressing so hard on her head that she is about to be embedded in the floor.

Then there's the question of the brushes. There are about twenty, and they all look more or less the same. Do I blend the foundation with a sponge or my fingers? I know from having interviewed many make-up artists that no two can agree on this anyway, so this doesn't worry me too much, but how do I know if I've put enough on? I find myself unconsciously mimicking what I've seen in photographic studios. It's a bit like having watched the safety demonstration on a plane a million times, then being asked to re-enact it – I can remember the bit about the oxygen mask, but not about taking my high-heeled shoes off before going down the chute.

The strange thing is that the things I expected to be difficult are actually easier than the things I thought were straightforward. Believe it or not, my *bête noire* – getting eyeliner on straight, is easier than blending a small isoceles-shaped triangle of black eyeshadow into the brown shadow on the upper lid. I am so absorbed in what I am doing that I forget what happens next. Is this the bit where the powder goes over the liner?

Rossi chats intermittently as she does the rounds, offering guidance and answering questions. 'Don't rub too hard,' she scolds. 'It'll make your work more difficult, as well as pulling the eyes of your model. Work the colour into the socket and up to the eyebrow, and remember, if you don't put too much on, you won't have so much blending to do.

'If you were doing this look on twelve girls for a show, you'd adapt it slightly according to the skin tone. Darker girls would have more black mixed into the brown eyeshadow.

'When you're on a shoot using a pencil inside the lower lid, always check through the camera. The heat of the lights can melt the line quickly and it can run.

'All of you have a lazy eye! I have to point things out that you should have seen yourself.' I am reminded of Barbara's comments about always looking.

While I am looking, I discover something I never knew before as I apply Julie's mascara. Our eyelashes are in two layers, one on top of the other! I know, it's fascinating, isn't it, but I always thought they were in one long layer, like false lashes. How could I have reached thirty-four years of age without discovering this? Lashes, when you look down on them, are so pretty. And while I am having this little private revelation, I am busted. 'I remember!' says Rossi. 'I met Kathleen when she used to be a model. We did some test shots together, and they were really nice! I am sure I still have them somewhere! You know, I never forget a face.' And the whole class looks at me, with, I swear, the exact look I was dreading: *She doesn't look like a model.*

TEN MINUTES ON THE PHONE WITH SOMEONE WHO DOES LOOK LIKE A MODEL: CHRISTY TURLINGTON

Christy was the model we all wanted to be. Half-Latin, of all the supermodels, she looked like she'd be the smartest, the nicest and the one who would most likely succeed in business, were there such a thing as a Supermodel Year Book.

How did you fit in to the world of make-believe?
'I started modelling at fifteen, and I stopped doing catwalks at twenty-five. Runway was torture. The media hype about it was the worst part. It's a lonely profession, and you work with groups of friends. It should be a time to build relationships because it is a bit like dormitory life. But once the media hype started, you couldn't really share a conversation with anyone. There were so many people who were so invasive, you'd see pictures that had nothing to do with the shows . . . we were just celebrity fodder.'

How did growing up in this industry affect your perception of beauty?

'When I started it was very different – at least in terms of what teenage models are exposed to today. It was all completely fluke. I didn't have any ideas about beauty, I didn't read magazines at all, so in a weird way, modelling was actually confidence-building. People in my industry like the odd proportions, the gangly bits. Growing up, I did start to see how so much focus on physical things could be dangerous – I heard about how people are influenced, but most young models don't really know who they are, or understand how they look could possibly have a negative influence on someone else.

'Airbrushing now is so out of control – I never did get used to that. I'm thirty-three now, and I don't need to be airbrushed under my eyes. Art directors want to feel like they have touched the image, and had some kind of manipulative influence. Beauty is about the moment, it is spontaneous, and that gets lost in the manipulation. Sometimes I could hardly relate to an image of myself on a billboard, because it wasn't me at all by the time it was finished. On the other hand, it was always very important to keep my family, friends and everything else separate. The industry – fashion and beauty – is fun; the travelling was exciting. It's not always superficial – there are a lot of genuine and very wonderful people, but the technology aspect has made that desire for perfection all the more dangerous.

'Now my company [she co-owns the ayurveda-based skincare line Sundari, as well as Nuala sportswear] is really based on the way you feel inside. I am very unmoved by physical beauty – we believe your skin and your face should exude the health and happiness from within.'

What was the best beauty tip you learnt from modelling?

That less is more. The stuff that has dated quickly is the more eccentric make-up. I also learned little things, like curling your lashes, instead of just putting mascara on.

When someone takes your picture now, do you go on auto-pilot?

'I don't think anyone likes having their picture taken. It's now only about twenty times a year, and actually, it's quite a nice break from the office.'

THE THREE MOST COMMON MAKE-UP MISTAKES ACCORDING TO BARBARA DALY

1 Applying make-up in bad light. 'It probably contributes more to people not getting their make-up right than any other single factor.'

2 Getting stuck in a make-up rut. To be wearing the same make-up you wore ten or fifteen years ago, or a version of it, is something that needs to be looked at. Find out how to change it, talk to an expert.

3 Buying the wrong shade of foundation. If in doubt, go lighter. What happens is you tend to make the purchase almost immediately in lighting circumstances that are not necessarily the best for choosing a foundation. If you're in a department store, take it to a window and use a hand mirror. Feel the texture on your hand, then blend it into your jawline. You shouldn't see anything there. A good foundation is one that will make people say, 'Hasn't she got great skin?' rather than 'What a great foundation.'

BARBARA DALY'S LOOK THAT WILL SUIT ANYONE – IN A FEW MINUTES

Learn to use a blusher. You can put it on your cheeks, lips and eyes for a mono-chromatic browny-pink look, then finish with a little bit of gloss, face powder and mascara. This is a modern look that looks great if you're sixteen or sixty. It goes with most fashions and you can do it in a few minutes.

MAKE ME OVER – NOW

If you are stuck in a make-up rut, or just want your make-up done before you go out, don't dismiss the assistants serving at make-up counters in department stores. They've come a long way from the white coats and orange faces they used to have. Many consultants are trained make-up artists, especially those at the more make-up-artist-geared brands, such as MAC, Nars, Shu Uemura or

Make Up For Ever. Usually the service is free, and often you don't need to book an appointment. If you're dining at eight, and finish work at six, it's a great way to kill time while feeling slightly pampered.

MAKE-UP AND AGEING: WHAT SUITS AND WHAT DOESN'T

- A hard lipline will age you more than a soft tinted lipstain.
- Creamy eyeshadow sits more easily on creased lids than powder. Keep the attention on the upper eyelids – apply a touch of white under the brows, and avoid eyeshadow and mascara on the bottom lashes.
- Eyebrow pencil that is too dark will make you look harder and older.
- A cream-textured blusher will deflect attention from crow's feet, but avoid anything that is too dark or contrasting, which will be harsh.
- And don't attempt to 'sculpt' your blusher – it is instantly ageing.

MAKE-UP KIT: THE MINIMUM TOOLS YOU NEED

- 1 natural sponge, to apply foundation with. 'You get a smoother finish with a natural sponge, used damp,' says Rossi. 'Wash it in washing-up liquid after every use.'
- 1 big powder brush, preferably goat's hair (it is stiffer than sable, so is easier to apply the powder with)
- 1 powder puff, to finish the powder with
- 1 round brush (sable) for the blusher. 'If you want to do some shading under the cheeks, a slanted brush is easier, though not strictly necessary.'
- 1 fairly large blending brush (sable) for the eyes
- 1 smaller eye brush (sable) for details on the eyes
- 1 medium brush (sable) to apply eyeshadow
- 1 pair of eyelash curlers, especially if your lashes are straight
- 1 small comb to separate the lashes after applying mascara (but before the mascara has dried)

- 1 old mascara brush to comb the eyebrows
- 1 lipbrush

DOWNSIZING MAKE-UP: WHAT YOU REALLY NEED

According to Glauca Rossi, apart from foundation, a good make-up kit should contain:

- 1 brown eyeshadow – 'You can wear it anywhere and with anything.'
- 1 black eyeshadow – 'You can use it in place of an eyeliner for a soft finish with a small brush.'
- 1 white or off-white eyeshadow to highlight under the browbone
- 1 coral-coloured blush
- 1 neutral, browny-pink lip colour – 'It suits everyone.'
- 1 good mascara, in either dark brown or black

HOW TO APPLY FOUNDATION AND CONCEALER – PART ONE: GLAUCA ROSSI

'The best way to apply foundation is by using a natural sponge. Dampen it, squeeze all the water out, then put the foundation on the back of your hand and start from the middle of the face, working your way outwards so you don't have any clogging near the hairline. Work your way down under the jawline, blending all the time. When you apply it to the forehead, put it on in the middle, and go up and out, blending carefully. Apply it under the eyes, over the eyes, you put it everywhere . . .

'It doesn't make sense to apply concealer first, because then when you blend it, it all comes off – I never understood why people did that,' says Glauca. 'Use your fingers, or even a brush if your concealer comes in a stick. Blend it out and down into the foundation so you don't have a line.'

WHAT ARE CORRECTIVE COLOURS?

These counteract any pigmentation problems. A green will take away the red tones of your skin. A pink or orange will take away the green. White will clarify and give a glow to your skin. 'You apply them before the foundation,' says Rossi. 'If you apply green over the foundation you will look like a Martian.'

GLAUCA ROSSI'S BROWN-EYED LOOK

This is the look I had to create in Rossi's lesson. Want to know how to do it? 'It was just one brown eye colour,' says Rossi, matter-of-factly. 'I blended towards the eyebrow and it faded.'

I promise you, it seemed much more complicated at the time.

COUNTER-CULTURE

A quick chat with the girls from Nars cosmetics, the make-up line by make-up artist François Nars, revealed the following:

- *The biggest mistake we make is choosing our foundation.*
- *We buy products we read about in magazines.*
- *Sometimes we need persuading to try colours that are out of our normal spectrum of greys and browns.*
- *We will buy things we've read that a celebrity uses.*
- *The best thing we can do for ourselves is to invest in a good set of brushes – 'They make application so much easier.'*
- *The best thing about working on the counter is 'making women feel happy about the way they look, and giving them the confidence to do it themselves'.*
- *The worst thing is 'Standing on our feet all day long'.*

What do real models really look like? Gorgeous. You want me to say, 'They're really ugly in real life, and incredibly stupid,' but sadly they're neither. They're worldly, switched on, and take their looks seriously, which is why they all drink so much water (removes toxins' etc.) and chain-smoke (that way you eat less food). Don't expect to relate to them physically, except the quirkier ones that is. That's another reason why the shows are relevant – as a token gesture, a reminder that beauty is about the individual after all. Not all girls look like Gisele or Cindy Crawford.

Occasionally, this individuality presents the make-up artist with problems, and that's where us mere mortals step in. One model's problems are an ordinary person's gain. Deep-set eyes? They've done them. Apply a light concealer with a pinky-peach tone to avoid the skin taking on a greyish pallor. No cheekbones to speak of? Avoid dark blusher, and keep the skin looking dewy and luminous. Put moisturiser under your blusher. Shiny skin? Beware of over-powdering – it looks just as bad as under-powdering. Thin lips? Avoid dark lipstick. Use blusher on your cheeks and accentuate your eyes, and if you're wearing lipstick, use a lipliner in the same colour to carefully, *carefully*, accentuate your lipline. What if you're just really old and craggy? Avoid foundation and powder, especially if your skin is very crêpey, and keep skin well moisturised. It does make fine surface lines disappear.

Nobody, not even a model, is perfect. 'There is a huge [and by huge, I am prepared to bet good money she means in terms of fame and not dress size] model, whose eyes are far, far too close together,' says Kay Montano, the make-up artist behind some of the most influential advertising campaigns and magazine visuals of the last ten years or so. We are sitting in the Westbourne pub, the restaurant co-owned by my husband Olly, me with my laptop, eating lunch and talking about make-up, waiting for my two-and-a-half-year-old son to turn up. (With his nanny, of course – I try not to encourage him to go to pubs by himself.) I first met Kay through Olly; they have been friends for years, and she has always been brilliant at returning calls on anything to do with work and make-up – like most in the business, she is professional at every level.

Kay is trying to convince me that the biggest flaws can be concealed, or at least improved, with make-up. 'Everything with make-up is an optical illusion,' she says. 'The key rule is simple enough: where there is darkness, you create light.' I put my soup spoon down temporarily and prepare to type away again. This sounds good. Only one rule!

'Think about it,' she says. 'Anything dark will sink in, or recede, whereas anything light stands out.' In other words, darkness under the eyes will disappear with a light-coloured concealer; and cheekbones will look more defined with a slightly shimmery blusher on top.

Kay's career started by accident. 'I was at school and had a friend who ended up wearing exactly the same clothes as me. We were both into the band Haysee Fantasee and had dreadlocks, everything in their style. We were horrible adolescents – we used to do things like steal wheelchairs from hospitals and spray them silver.'

'Why did you do that?'

'I don't know! We were just horrible!' she says. 'Then one day my friend met Kate Garner from the band [Kate later went on to become a successful video director], and we ended up hanging out with her. She said, "What do you want to do, Kay?" It just so happened that that week I wanted to be a make-up artist. She said, "Go and see Jamie Morgan," who was a photographer and a friend of hers, and I walked straight into that whole Buffalo scene. My first job, aged sixteen, was the front cover of *The Face*, styled by the late Ray Petri, with Nick Kamen modelling. Youth has tremendous power, I see that now.'

'Didn't you panic? How did you know what to do?'

'I did know a bit about make-up, because I used to look at *Cosmo* when I was fourteen and retouch their covers. I was obsessed. I didn't realise I was doing it – I'd be on the phone retouching eyelashes, putting on more lipstick . . . My mum bought me my first *Vogue*, and I still remember that Talisa Soto shoot by Bruce Weber. I knew every model, and I'd copy the make-up on myself. I was so heavy-handed – I wore really thick base when I had perfect skin.'

Now she is based in New York, although her home is London. A typical day has her turning up at a studio with a rough outline of the day ahead. She'll know the photographer, the fashion editor and perhaps the model. 'If it's a specialist thing, then I will be told to bring specific make-up. Normally I'm always prepared, though. I have a big kit.'

It can be every bit as glamorous as we imagine it to be. 'Doing big celebs is really glamorous. Nicole Kidman, Cameron Diaz . . . they are all lovely and they wouldn't be where they are without being that way. The most glamorous job I ever did? I remember doing the campaign for Calvin Klein Obsession with Kate Moss and being flown to Virgin Gorda,' she says. 'They knew they wouldn't need any make-up at all, but they flew me out just in case. In the end they used the pictures Mario Sorrenti, the photographer, and Kate's boyfriend at the time, shot before we got there. He had wanted to create the feeling of intimacy, so he didn't want me or Drew (Jarrett, the hairstylist) to be on the set at the time. That whole trip, the hardest thing I had to think about was what kind of sunblock I would need.'

Her most unusual job was going to No. 10 to do John Major's grooming and Norma's make-up. 'It was so surreal!' she laughs. 'I was in their bedroom and I could see what kind of books they read and that they had a horrible-looking fireplace, and I kept thinking, "This is so weird! it's like a bad hotel!" I had that Sex Pistols song going round and round my head . . . "Anarchy in the UK" . . . But they were so charming, very charming.'

The downside is less obvious. 'You have to always act as if you're the happiest person in the world, regardless of whether you have just split up with your boyfriend, or if you feel sick. You are constantly on audition – every job is with new people. I have to be Mum all the time. Every day is your first day at work – you got that job over ten other equally brilliant people. It is a lot of pressure, and sometimes that can tip you over the edge. Your private life is practically impossible – you just cannot have a long-term relationship in the business until you are really, really well known. Most of the time you fly economy, and go straight to work . . .'

It's also a very different world to the one in which she started all those years ago. 'Now, if you worked for *The Face* with someone of Ray Petri's calibre, you'd immediately be doing the next Balenciaga campaign,' says Kay. 'In those days, the fashion brands didn't understand "street" fashion. It was much more about music, hip hop, rap . . . It was a sub-culture. After a point I realised there was nothing sophisticated about my work, and I went off to Paris to work for fashion magazines there. When I came back to London I was still only eighteen, but suddenly I was taken seriously and started working for *Vogue*.'

The irony of it all is that although Kay has been responsible for creating looks that are at the same time directional, visually exciting and beautiful, her favourite look is – natural. 'I do think the catwalk is still relevant,' she says. 'The first time you see things it is always shocking. But it's not meant to be taken literally. You have to remember these people are selling a black dress to the public twice a year – it's bound to be fickle. How else do you make it constantly seem interesting? My style, I suppose, is to bring out the strengths of each person, which is why I love working with actresses, to hear about their experiences and to see the way they convey emotion. I approach every face absolutely differently. One look does not suit all.'

Make-up artist Charlotte Tilbury agrees – and, let's face it, it's not rocket science to figure it out, but it does make a nonsense of all those books with precise painting-by-numbers diagrams of how to apply make-up, unless you know how to adapt their step-by-steps to suit you and your hooked nose/blotchy skin/warty eyelids/whatever. You need to know your own face before you attempt any major changes. 'Some people have an artistic flare, and some people are very good at doing their own make-up, but the majority of people haven't got a bloody clue,' Tilbury says. We are in another local restaurant, and this time I have my dictaphone on the table. Occasionally people at the surrounding tables look up and glance at her. She must be a film star, or someone very important, otherwise why would she be being inter-viewed? She does look a little like a film star, it has to be said. She arrives forty minutes late, just like a film star, and gushes her hellos, kissing me on each cheek. She has lots of flame red hair, the palest of skins, tight black trousers and high heels. Ten minutes with Tilbury is like a weekend in New York – you're left with your head spinning, re-energised and wanting more, more, more of everything.

For now, I just want more about make-up. 'People don't know how to dissect their faces. They know themselves so well because they're looking in the mirror every day, but they can't look in a deconstructive way,' she continues. 'Whereas when I stand in front of someone I look at their face and think, okay, their eyes are too close together, their eyebrows need sharpening up, they need to widen this section of the face or plump up this section, they should narrow this . . .'

Have you ever tried eating lunch with a make-up artist? At this precise point all I can think about is, 'Why didn't I pluck my eyebrows? Is my concealer blended correctly? Do I have too much blusher on?' This is one of the rare occasions I have actually bothered to put make-up on. I did it for Tilbury's sake. And I'm now worried I might have got it wrong.

'You see with you,' she continues, 'I would probably bring your eyes out slightly because they're deep-set, but also I'd make the most of that fact and try to make them a little bit harem-y. I'd line them. I'd go with what your assets are, rimming the eyes with a chocolate black/brown liner, blending it out at the edges. Very Salma Hayek.'

'I wouldn't look like a panda?'

'You'd need some concealer to cover the shadows and maybe don't bring down the eyeliner too low, so you still have that feline look, but it's definitely a cat not a panda.'

'You know,' she continues (focusing her gaze somewhere around my forehead), 'I don't think people take enough care of their eyebrows. They don't understand, these are the pillars of the face! They will make you look sad, they'll make you look sleepy, they'll make you look untidy, and, if you fix them, they will completely transform you. Also, the colour of the eyebrow. Some blondes, for example, because they have dyed their hair are naturally blessed with darker brows. But a lot of blondes are a bit too fair, or they're too washed out, and their eyebrows should be dyed. I mean, I'm an albino without dyeing mine. You wouldn't recognise me, because I don't have a face. It's all washed out.'

She goes on to tell me that you should get your brows dyed professionally. The colour is left on for perhaps half a minute and then taken off. It has to be done gradually or by someone who really knows your natural colour, otherwise you end up looking like two big fat caterpillars have been glued to your face.

Lashes are perhaps the next most important thing, to Tilbury at least. Hers are heavily mascara'd. In her book you can never have too much of it, especially if it's over curled or even permed lashes – Kate Moss, incidentally, is a big fan of perming. In my book, which is this one, you can have too much mascara. Big, clumpy lashes are great – I love them – but just be aware that that's the look you're going for. Otherwise, get the comb out and comb them through while they're still wet, like the rest of us. Tilbury even puts her mascara on first, before the rest of make-up. She says it gives a more defined look if you're fair, making it easier to follow the shape of the eyes when applying an eyeliner.

'Mascara really wakes up the whole eye area. It gives your eyes a sexier look, rather than this canopy, which can make the eye look hooded and half asleep. I really feel that eyebrows and eyelashes are something you can do without having to put on make-up every day, and they can totally transform a face. And the eyes, at the end of the day – without sounding like too much of a major hippy – are the windows to your soul.' She's right. I have seen this happen with my own face. Years fly off you. People tell you how well you look. And it's all because a few stray hairs have been removed from that space between the eyes.

Tilbury has moved on now: 'Do you fancy checking out Portobello market this afternoon? Kate Moss had on this fantastic fake fur coat the other day, and she says there are loads of them under the archway on the left . . .'

AND NOW, WOMEN OF COLOUR, LET ME INTRODUCE YOU TO ATEH DAMACHI

Ateh is the beauty assistant at *Tatler* and always arrives at the office glowing, with perfectly applied make-up. But it wasn't always so well applied. Her mother is from Trinidad and her father from Nigeria, and she remembers having some pretty terrifying make-up experiences as a teenager. Anyway, I'll let Ateh tell you all about it.

'When I was fourteen, I wanted to buy some make-up product or other that all my friends would buy, and I remember walking into a department store and finding the whole thing totally horrendous. There were rows and rows of foundations, all in shades of rose through to beige – if you were lucky. Everything was ashy – I really don't know who those colours were meant to suit. I felt so excluded, and I remember thinking, "They're telling me I can't be beautiful" – that's quite difficult for a sensitive fourteen-year-old to get her head around. Then I discovered MAC, which was a really good step in the right direction because the coloured pigments in the eyeshadows were a lot stronger, so they would show up on my dark skin. They did have black foundations – a limited number – and they were good – nowhere near what they have today, but in terms of texture and finish, it was there. My skin has blue undertones – other parts have yellow undertones – so what I do now with my foundation is only apply it where I need it, and mix it first with an iridescent moisturiser to give my skin a glow. What is still really annoying is that I cannot think of a nice compact or loose powder in one of the cheaper mass-market lines. On one magazine I worked on, I would say that 60 per cent of the phone enquiries we had were from women with Asian skins who couldn't find the right coloured concealer. They were more for bronzed skins than Asian skin.

'The ideal look for me is a lovely nude look. People see black skins and they attack you with purple! But no, I want to look fresh, pretty and natural, like I've just been nibbling cherries like everyone else . . .'

'TOM PECHEUX' SMOKY EYES IN FIVE MINUTES

Apply mascara on your upper and lower lids, then put black pencil on the inside of the eyes, smudging it a little. Keep your lips matt with a beige colour. I thought this was so easy, I stole it from an earlier interview I did with Tom Pecheux in *Tatler*.

WHAT ANNOYS KAY MONTANO

1   Using bad fake tans.
2   Using liners that have nothing to do with the colour of our lips. 'America has a big problem with lipliner.'
3   Overplucking our eyebrows.

KAY MONTANO'S SMOKY EYE – FOR WHEN YOU HAVE A LITTLE MORE TIME

The smoky eye and natural lip is a classic, but it doesn't suit everyone. Very few older women can get away with it. Make sure your skin is blemish-free, but not heavily covered, otherwise it can look too much like a mask. After applying a light base, take a brown eye pencil and draw a soft, wide line next to your top lashes, keeping it broader at the outside edge and narrower in the corner. (Start from the corner or the middle of the eyelid, whatever's easier.) Using a fat eyeshadow brush, blend the line in. On top of this, apply a taupe/grey eyeshadow with a little bit of pearl, which helps prevent the eye from looking too gothic. Using the large brush again, blend deeper into the eye socket and right across the eyelid. (Brushes are really important: you do need a big eyeshadow brush – that is the key to getting it soft, not hard.) The colour must go in an upward direction, not downwards, otherwise it drags the whole eye down. Then, take a sharpened black eye pencil and draw a fine line next to your upper lashes. If your eyes can take it, you can use a small eyeshadow brush to blend a little bit under your eyes next to your lashes. (If your eyes droop downwards, they can't take this, and it's not a good look for overly round eyes either.) Use eyelash curlers on the top lashes and finish with lots and lots of black mascara and a transparent beige or neutral gloss on the lips.

HOW TO LOOK INSTANTLY GLAMOROUS

'Invest in some good eyelash curlers,' says Kay Montano. 'There is something about curled eyelashes and mascara which really opens up the eye and makes you look bright and alert. Whenever I want to look glam I'll make sure my eyelashes look really "worked".'

HOW TO PAINT THE PERFECT PLUM LIPS

Apply the lip colour using a brush. Soften the line with a cotton bud, and blot it a few times. Reapply, then blot. Keep skin really natural, but with a cream blusher on your cheeks in a similar plum colour, and a little mascara to finish.

Why do most make-up artists hardly wear make-up themselves?

'Because they're like most women. They just don't wear very much,' says Kay Montano. 'A blusher, eyelash curlers, tinted gloss and mascara . . . It's not really keeping the make-up companies in business, is it?'

HOW TO APPLY FOUNDATION – PARTS TWO AND THREE: KAY MONTANO AND CHARLOTTE TILBURY

Something you would think is so simple is actually quite complicated – make-up artists all seem to have different ways of applying foundation. Kay Montano applies it by mixing foundation with a moisturiser that suits the person's skin type, e.g. if you have oily skin, mix a moisturiser for oily skins with foundation in equal parts. Use a sponge to apply it, blending as you go along. There should be nothing left by the time you get to the jaw. Charlotte Tilbury prefers to use fingers – 'You can work the foundation into the skin and you get a dewy effect, whereas I find that sponges retain too much and leave a film between you and the skin so it's harder to make it look natural. Powders these days can be like silk – dust them on, especially over the T-zone, using a big brush. Tap the powder brush on your wrist first to remove the excess. Never cake on too much. And only ever apply your foundation and cover-up to areas that need it. You don't need to do a whole face – try and leave as much of your good skin on show as possible.'

BRUSH, SPONGE OR FINGERS, FOR CONCEALER?

Use a brush for greater precision.

EYELASHES – YOU'RE NOT READY FOR THE PERM YET

And why would you be, when you can warm up a pair of metal eyelash curlers with a hairdryer for a few seconds, apply them as usual to your lashes, and achieve the same effect, if not better?

EYEBROW PLUCKERS: THROW THOSE TWEEZERS AWAY, HERE'S KAMINI VAGHELA, THE THREADER

Threading is a technique for hair removal that originated in Asia. It's a real skill and, unfortunately, it's hard to find people who are experienced enough to do it, and who have the eye to tell how much of the eyebrow to trim, and how much to leave alone – although this goes for plucking as well.

'I look at the whole face, see what the original shape of the brow is, and decide how to enhance and perfect it,' says Vaghela. The process is quite extraordinary. She takes a cotton thread, knots it as if about to do a cat's cradle, and then grips one individual hair between the threads. She twists and slides the thread, and then pulls it without raising the skin, and out comes the hair. Her dexterous hands move fast. It's gentler than plucking, and the whole process is over in about ten minutes.

The advantages of threading are that the hairs grow back softer, and usually in a natural direction, so when you've had it done once it's easier to maintain the shape. Vaghela has a good eye: she realised that previous pluckers had inadvertently shortened the ends of mine – she's now elongated them, just by letting the ones at the end grow back.

The disadvantages are that you need to be in the right hands, and it's a technique not many people can do. Overplucking and breaking the hairs off instead of pulling them out from the root are two big eyebrow crimes.

If you can't get them threaded, avoid waxing at all costs – it's much harder for the therapist to get a precise shape.

WHAT'S FASHIONABLE IN EYEBROWS NOW?

Whatever suits your face. This is one example of how misleading fashion can be. Eyebrows are totally about bone structure. True, you can leave them to grow a bit thicker once in a while, but radical trends are best avoided unless you want to look completely and utterly ridiculous.

WHAT TO DO WHEN YOU HAVE OVERPLUCKED YOUR EYEBROWS

Believe it or not, supermodel Gisele has eyebrows that are too close together and need bringing out. 'I use an eyeshadow and eye pencil,' says Charlotte Tilbury. 'I draw the line. We make the eyebrow shape stronger to follow the eyes, arching, lifting them up and bringing them out. Even when she's wearing no make-up, we'll do this to her eyes, and it makes a massive difference.' There's hope for us all then.

WHAT ANNOYS CHARLOTTE?

Charlotte Tilbury says: Harsh lipliners, the kind that are one or two shades darker than your main lip colour, are a big no-no. 'They're old, ageing, and not fresh or modern.'

CHARLOTTE TILBURY'S BRIGITTE BARDOT

'You should only take elements of Brigitte, otherwise you'll look ridiculous. Use a cream eyeshadow in brown or grey. Blend a little into the eye socket. Line your eyes with black or brown, depending on whether you're fair or dark. Blend the socket line out in an upwards direction towards the brow – but not too much. The aim is to make your eyes look bigger and doe-like, sexy and slanty. Innocent and helpless but also, "I'm really naughty". Put lashes and lashes of mascara on. Finish with a little bit of natural lip gloss, or blend it in with a lipliner.'

CHARLOTTE TILBURY'S CHARLOTTE RAMPLING

'Red lips. Very sexy. Nothing else. It's a classic. If you have smaller lips, use a little lipliner, then, using a brush, go over it with the red lipstick, otherwise skip the lipliner. Blot the lipstick with a tissue, apply a light dusting of powder with a puff, then reapply the lipstick. Finish with just a touch of mascara.'

CHARLOTTE TILBURY'S GISELE (THE MODEL, NOT THE BALLET)

'Use a bronzer or fake tan that is absorbed as much as possible by the skin, like a mousse or a gel – nothing that sits on top of the skin like a foundation. Put it on a cotton pad and rub it all over your face for an instant brown glow. If you're really pale, just apply it across the bridge of the nose where the sun would naturally hit, along the cheekbones, on the temples and on the chin. If you're a bit darker, you can use a bronzing powder to finish. Enhance the natural pigment colour of your lips with lipstain in pinks, pale reds, essences of terracotta. It gives you the kind of look you last had when you were eight and spent some time by the seaside. Apply a cream blush in the same kind of colour over the cheekbones and on the bridge of the nose – put some also on the eyes. Use an eye pencil that has a bit of bronze or gold in it all the way around the eyes, and, if you're brave, apply a touch of eye gloss – use Vaseline or a specialist make-up brand. Mascara, naturally, is the final touch.'

CHARLOTTE TILBURY'S CARRIE FROM SEX AND THE CITY

'She wears the same make-up all the way through. She wears a little bit of powder. I'd say that she uses a cream blush, leaving a light sheen. Powder down the T-zone to get rid of excess grease. On the eyes she uses a silvery-grey colour with a slight sheen. Apply a charcoal grey pencil inside the eye, then a dove grey slightly underneath. Use lots of mascara on the bottom and top lashes. Use a lip pencil, but work it in very naturally with a shimmery lip gloss on top. Choose a rose-pink colour. I don't know who does the make-up for that programme, but they've set a trend all the way around the world. It's fresh, girly, naughty. Big pink cheeks, pretty pink lips . . . it takes the hardness off her face.'

CHARLOTTE TILBURY'S BIG BEAUTY SECRET

'Basically you have to look gorgeous the whole time. Although I do now let my boyfriend see me with no eyelashes, it did take four years. You should always have a little bit of mystery, always look a bit gorgeous, always look a little bit fetching in the morning. And never let a man know about your beauty secrets.' For a moment, I thought I was talking to the late Barbara Cartland, but no, Tilbury is deadly serious. She's not the only one – I even know of one famous female pop star who has told me she jumps out of bed ten minutes before her boyfriend wakes up to repair her face. I'm not saying who because she'd kill me.

Every make-up artist's dream product: Touche Éclat (Radiant Touch) by Yves Saint-Laurent, a concealer that isn't a concealer but a light-reflecting wand of magic. How did Terry de Gunzberg create it?

'It was a combination of three things I would do when working as a make-up artist in shows with models,' says Terry, who created the make-up for YSL for over twenty years, as well as developing her own line, By Terry. 'I wanted to refresh, to add a glow, without any extra coverage. I would mix on the back of my hands a drop of toner, a drop of moisturiser and a drop of very light foundation. I'd apply it under the eyes with a flat brush and in the curves of the face, and then I'd blend it with my fingertips to revamp the existing make-up. I used this technique for twenty-five years. At the time I was creating the cosmetics for Yves Saint-Laurent. I asked the laboratory if they could blend these three dimensions so I wouldn't have to make it myself each time – it was very difficult to find the right balance between coverage, light and the feeling of having bare skin. It then took me another three years to convince the management to launch the products because no one wanted to accept the idea of one single colour for a universal market. So I decided to take this product and go on a tour worldwide to present it myself to the beauty editors. And, of course, they knew straight away what it was about because they're cleverer than the people in the industry. Now a lot of people know about Touche Éclat and they don't even know it's by YSL. And I'm working on a new updated version for my own cosmetic line, By Terry.'

MAKE-UPOLOGY: WHAT DOES IT ALL MEAN?

Highlighter: This should go from the end of the browbone to the cheekbone, to highlight the cheekbone.

Pigment: This is a micro-prism of synthetic or mineral particles, or natural particles from pearls or other ingredients. They are different shapes, sometimes luminous, and can reflect light and generate a colour.

Socket line: It's where you can feel the ball of your eye – in between the brow-bone and the ball.

'What's the point of getting your hair cut? It only grows again.'
attrib Alphonse Allais, French humourist
(1854–1905),

'And all the time, I was dancing round that small, blonde head, snipping here, flicking a comb there . . . while the flashbulbs popped and the jazz band played . . .'
Vidal Sassoon on cutting Mia Farrow's hair
(Sorry I Kept You Waiting Madam, Cassell, 1968)

Chapter Four

ALL HAIL EUGENE THE KING!

Getting a haircut is a life-changing event. When I die, instead of my life flashing before me, I expect to be reminded of the Mary Quant bob aged three, the Nana Mouskouri impersonator aged eight; the too-short fringe that prompted classmates to pin up tribal pictures from *National Geographic* on my locker door; the Flock of Seagulls shaved sides and spiky top from my late teen period; and the final exhibit: today's J-Lo on a good day, cable TV weather girl on a bad day (pre-Ulrika Jonssen, neatly parted to avoid the outcrop of grey springing up where once I had a side parting).

My present dissatisfaction with the way I look has no bearing on the hairstyle whatsoever (which actually, isn't that bad), but is more to do with the fact that I have committed the cardinal sin of diverting from type. Because you're either a long-haired woman or a short-haired one, it's as simple as that. You can dabble with a cut, a fringe, or try growing it for a while, but sooner or later, you'll revert to the pre-destined gene that dictates all women's hairstyles.

Long versus short has nothing to do with age, either. It used to be the saying that any woman over thirty should cut off her long hair or risk looking like mutton dressed as lamb. Many of today's hair heroines, frequently over thirty, have sensibly ignored this advice, with the result that several 'most requested hairstyles' belong to women like Elizabeth Hurley, Nigella Lawson and Yasmin Le Bon. They're popular because, unlike the classic TV commercials for Salon Selectives shampoos, these are women who *don't* look like 'they just stepped out of a salon'.

But, casual as these styles look, you can bet that hours will have gone into achieving them. Behind every successful woman is a great hairdresser. There is also a great communicator. Being able to explain exactly what you want is half of the challenge. I have spent hours in a salon only to emerge looking exactly the same – because 'Something natural, yet a bit brighter please' was interpreted as 'maintenance'. Like most beauty editors, incidentally, I get my haircuts for free, so I put it all down to experience and wait until next time, but if I'd been paying the £200 or so it costs to see one of the top stylists, I might have tried a bit harder to say something more worthwhile.

So what makes a great haircut? Versatility, perhaps? Being able to do things with it? Catwalk shows are a real testing ground for whether a model has a versatile look or not. Hairdressers have to work with all sorts, and the 'star' hairdresser has to draw on the experience of a carefully selected team of anything from ten to thirty assistants to help him or her achieve something worthy of the world's assembled fashion press waiting impatiently outside. Models have been known to turn up with glue in their hair – the remains of extensions used in previous shows. If their hair is too stylised – a Peggy Moffat bob, for example, might be fine for certain shows, but not for others – hairpieces, dyed to match the exact shade of the model's own hair have to be seamlessly attached.

It always amazes me that working in such conditions, a top stylist will still have time to answer the annoying questions of pesky journalists such as myself, but, all credit to them, most do. Backstage at the Julien MacDonald show in London, Eugene Soulieman is shadowed by a queue of three, one of whom is me. When it's finally my turn, a long, lanky photographer strolls past and whispers something in Soulieman's ear, then laughs and walks away. 'What did he say?' I ask. 'All hail Eugene the king! . . . or something silly,' says Soulieman, as embarrassed as I am. An exaggeration, perhaps, but not entirely inappropriate. As far as hairdressers go, Soulieman is definitely up there with the best of them. He is incredibly charming, with a face that is crinkly, lived in, cheeky. In an instant he puts the final nail into the coffin of any myths of hairdressers wearing leather trousers – he's far too cool for any of that rubbish.

'I am not a grungy hairdresser,' he says, when I ask him how he would define his style. 'I like to do things that are well-crafted, flavourful, modern. Hairdos without the finish. Something that is perfect, but then played around with until it is slightly wrong. It's the attitude really.'

The creator of some of the most directional catwalk looks, he'll draw on references from the past – a David Bowie album cover, for example – but add his own stamp, working closely with the designer and the make-up artist for an overall look that also brings out the best of each model's features. He has some interesting techniques – at a previous show I found him stamping straightening irons over hair that in turn was folded over a knife to create a wave; at another, he was braiding the hair on the sides and fastening it tightly at the back with elastic bands to pull the sides of the face taut and make the eyes seem more expressive. Maybe this is what they mean by the lunch-time facelift.

But behind such showmanship are the skills that got him to this position in the first place – years of training and working under the Vidal Sassoon banner mean he can cut a classic five–point bob better than most stylists. This being a man who clearly knows about hair, it is reassuring to know that 'No particular cut is better to work with. In fact, I sometimes like it if it isn't perfect. Something else happens then, there is more energy.' Try telling that to your colleagues when you go into the office with a lop-sided fringe. And being able to comb it the other way isn't much compensation either. So much for versatility then. Yes, it's great to have a cut you can do things with, but what if you're not Eugene, or even a dab hand with a blow-dryer? Better to get the cut right from the start.

But which cut is the right cut? If he could narrow it down to three, hairdresser Charles Worthington – who has a salon in west London and a product range almost everywhere you look – would say the layered cut, the classic blunt one-length cut, and the graduated cut, are the only three you need to know about. 'Everything else is a combination of the above, adapted according to the tools you use – a razor instead of scissors, for example,' he says. Worthington is refreshingly frank and simplistic about his craft, and puts his success – and yours – in getting a great haircut down to, again, communication. He's rather good at communicating. He talks animatedly of a movie premiere he's just come back from in Los Angeles. Jennifer Aniston was sitting on his right; Rosanna Arquette on his left.

'America is all about celebs,' he says. 'You've just got to be doing them. UK celebs are no good either. Americans only want ones they've heard of.' Fortunately for him, Goldie Hawn was 'in last week', so he's never short of a name or two to drop. Fortunately for us, he's not just good at communicating with celebrities.

'Sixteen years ago, when we started this business, we decided to ensure our training programme placed equal emphasis on communication skills and craft skills,' he says. 'A good haircut is so important, because it's framing a picture, the picture being your face. It's not just about being technically perfect, it has to suit your face shape, your hair texture and your lifestyle. When these three things gel, that's a good haircut.'

You might feel a little silly tearing out a picture of Jennifer, Rosanna or Goldie before you visit a salon, but Worthington thinks it's a good idea to have some visual reference as it gives your stylist a pointer as to which direction you want to head for. Obviously you have to be a bit open-minded after that – it's not their fault if you don't leave looking exactly like your favourite film star – and every style needs to be interpreted into something that suits your face shape. All this should be discussed in a consultation, preferably a couple of days before your actual appointment, so you have time to go away and think about your style of choice.

How do you find a good hairdresser to talk to in the first place? Word of mouth is the way I've always found to be most successful, but if you don't find yourself coveting any of your friends' hairstyles, go to a salon where you like the look of the staff, book in for a consultation with a senior stylist and look for a positive attitude. If you don't want to bring along a picture, or no specific image springs to mind, ask to see a style book. And remember, according to Worthington: 'Too much negativity on the part of your stylist is often a way of disguising a lack of skill.' In other words, if they don't make you feel confident, go somewhere else.

NICKY CLARKE'S FIVE GOLDEN RULES OF GREAT HAIR

Hairdresser Nicky Clarke is a genius cutter – if ever you are lucky enough to sit in the hot seat at his grand mirrored Mayfair salon, flanked by his two assistants armed with their blow-dryers, you will be amazed at how fast and furious he can be with a pair of scissors, and how glamorous he can make your hair look in just forty-five minutes. Best of all, his mum brings his lunch, and that of this brother, fellow hairdresser Michael van Clarke, to their respective salons every day. (Aah!) Last time I was there he told me that whenever someone complains to him of a bad hair day, he knows it will be down to not following one of the five rules of great hair . . . which are:

1 Wash your hair properly. Using the right shampoo and conditioner and rinsing your hair thoroughly in warm, running water is the start of making your hair look great.

2 Get the best cut you can to suit your lifestyle, the fashions you like and your level of maintenance. Enhance what you have rather than going for radical changes.

3 Use the correct styling products. This doesn't have to mean overloading your hair with styling products – you're aiming to look as if you don't have anything in your hair at all – rather, using them intelligently. If you have fine hair use a thickening spray, mousse or gel, and if you have frizzy hair learn how to calm it down with products applied to the mid-lengths or ends of the hair.

4 Learn how to dry your hair correctly. It doesn't need to take hours, it might not even involve a hairdryer. Unless you are moving from one extreme type to another (e.g. trying to go from curly to straight hair), it should only take about fifteen minutes to blow-dry your hair. Dry it off until it is about 80 per

cent dry: the real work is in the remaining 20 per cent. A quick way to a lift at the roots when you don't have time to wash your hair, is to spray volumising spray on them. Spritz it on dry hair without drenching it, then put big velcro rollers in, and get in the bath or put your make-up on. That ten to fifteen-minute period is all it takes. You take the rollers out, turn your head upside down, brush it lightly, and you've got a bounce.

5 Don't forget the finishing details: you can have a straightforward haircut, but apply the right finishing product and you have a very different look, turning one cut into something with a different texture and finish.

TOP STYLES IN TEN MINUTES NO. 1: THE SLICKED-BACK PONYTAIL

Apply a serum to wet hair. Blow-dry with a paddle brush, getting it as straight as you can, using a nozzle on the dryer for more precision – it stops you from lifting the hair and blowing it about too much. (If you have curly hair, use a natural brush as this puts more tension in the hair and allows you to grip and pull the curl out more.) Smooth a small amount of wax over the surface to catch any stray hairs and pull back into a ponytail using a snag-free band, or a hook hair elastic.

A SHORT HISTORY OF MODERN HAIRDRESSING BY JOHN FRIEDA

'The hairdressing business really got going in the Fifties. My father was a hairdresser and I remember him talking a lot about people like Raymond in the UK, who was the first TV celebrity hairdresser, and was known as 'Mr Teasy Weasy'. I suppose his counterpart in Paris would have been Alexandre, who was famous for his glamorous styling. And then Vidal Sassoon came along, and the whole focus changed, from being about hairstyling – setting it in rollers, back-combing it, putting it up in elaborate chignons – to being all about cutting. Sassoon, who had trained with Raymond, among others, revolutionised everything. He said, 'No more rollers – just a cut and blow-dry.' The only thing you need is your scissors, a blow-dryer and a brush.' It was a very important statement because hairdressing moved from perming and curling to cutting precisely, geometrically. From the Sixties right through to the Seventies nobody had such an influence on the profession worldwide as he did. The Sandy Shaw, the three-point cuts . . . these were his inventions. But in other respects it could be limiting, and that's where Leonard came in.

'Leonard had been trained by Rose Evansky, one of the few really successful female hairdressers who knew how to dress hair beautifully. He also worked with Vidal, and was his top stylist. He opened his first salon in the Seventies, which is when I started working for him. He was brilliant, although people haven't heard of him in the same way as they have heard of Sassoon. He could cut hair incredibly well, but differently from Vidal. Whereas what Vidal was doing was all very geometric, Leonard was always looking at the face. He wasn't trying to create a work of art, he was considering the person underneath and would never do anything on a woman that wouldn't suit her. He worked with *Vogue* and had a tremendous influence, spawning so many great hairdressers . . . Michaeljohn, Bumble and Bumble, all these salons had their roots with him.

'As for now, it's the era of the session stylist, the people who create the looks on shoots and at shows. Orlando Pita is brilliant, with a great eye and a way of making the hair work with the clothes as well as being a really lovely guy. Odile Gilbert is from the French school, and very original. She did the Chanel shows for years and years. Sam McKnight is great, very skilled and always makes the girls look beautiful. Sally Hershberger is able to create looks that everyone wants, most famously Meg Ryan.'

What is John Frieda's most requested short hairstyle?
It belongs to his ex-wife, Lulu. Kiki Koh, a stylist in John Frieda's Mayfair salon, says he does up to five a day of her short, choppy, bob. 'I can spot them waiting in reception.'

Did I say 'John Frieda'?

Well, yes, I did, and now that we're on the subject, he is possibly the richest man in hairdressing, thanks to the clever invention of a product called Frizz-Ease, a smoothing serum which is the best-selling hair product in the USA. That, and the fact that he just sold his company for around US$450 million. Over tea at Claridges, he tells me how it was born.

'My business partner Gail Federici has always had frizzy hair. She said, "Look, I'm so typical of a lot of people with this hair type, and there is nothing out there that will solve it." So we talked to chemists and told them that we wanted something that would alter the surface texture of the hair and make it smooth without making it oily or greasy. And that was how we developed it. We launched in 1991 and we didn't have much money to advertise, so we needed something that really got the message across.' The ads, with a before and after picture of a girl with frizzy hair and then smooth hair, were so simple the message couldn't possibly be confused. 'That one product has influenced the whole industry.'

HOW TO BE BEAUTIFUL BY JOHN FRIEDA

'It's not the wrapping that's important, but it's what's inside once you open it up. Real beauty is not about great hair and make-up, although there's nothing wrong in trying to make the most of yourself. There are people who I don't think of as being anything other than completely and utterly beautiful just because they are really good, nice people.'

SAM McKNIGHT, THE HAIRDRESSERS' HAIRDRESSER, LOOKS BACK ON THE ICONIC STYLES OF THE LAST THREE DECADES

When I first met Sam McKnight I was nervous to say the least. I had flown over from Sydney, where I was beauty editor of *Marie Claire Australia* to do a shoot in New York with the photographer Josh Jordan. Sam was doing hair, and Mary Greenwell was doing make-up. Both were at the top of their professions. Both of them, by sheer virtue of being in a studio with me, were slumming it somewhat, and I'm really not trying to be self-deprecating when I say this. We needed them more than they needed us. I still need Sam more than he needs me, but fortunately he can always be coerced into contributing to articles I'm writing because he loves his job. Long may he stay loving it.

This is how he views the last three decades, in hair-styling terms at least.

'I've been styling hair for over twenty-five years. The business didn't really exist back then. I was working in Molton Brown and one day I got called in to take Kerry Warn's place on a job. I started doing *Vogue* in 1980. Of course, it can be incredibly glamorous. You can be on Concorde to New York, leaving at 10.30 in the morning and arriving two hours before you took off. You fly back straight after a day's work in the studio or at a show: let's not make any bones about it, this is a glamorous job! But you can also find yourself in the back of a Winnebago feeling sick because you've been driving for two hours out in the Mohave desert with people you don't particularly want to be with, having been up since 4 a.m. in order to catch the light - and you've still got to do the hair.

'In the early 80s none of us knew what was happening. The supermodel thing just exploded. It was all androgynous, street, post-punk, post-disco, post-New Romantic, and it was incredibly creative because the big money hadn't yet taken over. All the young designers, like Calvin Klein, John Galliano and Vivienne Westwood were still in their formative years. Magazines like *The Face* and *Vogue* fused music, the arts, street culture, and fashion into one thing, which had never really happened on a large scale before.

'In the early 80s, the hairstyle belonged to model **Jenny Howarth**. She was the muse of photographer Steven Meisel. She had a ginger, messy bob before, and had decided to stop modelling. We were having such a great time on the shoot, and decided to be really mischievous with her hair. We thought: ooh, what can we do to really destroy it! I cut her hair so short you could practically see her scalp through it, then we bleached it, planning to then dye it back to her own colour. It looked so great that we all cut our own hair off and bleached it blonde. The finished style - a short, androgynous cut – had a real impact and of course, it certainly didn't finish her career. It was totally anti that whole "just stepped out of a salon" thing. It was the beginning of another phase for her.'

Linda Evangelista was very much the look of the late 80s. 'She was another of Meisel's muses. She really was instrumental in making the whole business extremely glamorous because she had the ability to change her hair from long to short to blonde to ginger to black, and was very pro-active in how the pictures and images were made. Julien d'Ys cut her hair from long to short. It was a great hair cut. After Jenny's hair cut, the pendulum of fashion had swung from short to long, and suddenly it was all about Cindy Crawford and Yasmin Le Bon. What was great about Linda's cut was that it was another short hair style. It would still be wearable now.

'For the 90s it has to be **Kate Moss**. When I first met her she was a pretty little English girl on a go-see for a job with photographer Steven Klein. At the time everyone was photographing her as a grungy, skinny thing with stringy hair. I was working a lot with Vivienne Westwood at the time, and we put her in wigs. It was amazing to watch her metamorphose into this beautiful, really elegant creature. She used to scream at me, "DON'T PUT THOSE ROLLERS IN MY HAIR!" and complain that I'd make her look just like her mum, but in fact it only took a little bit of work to make her look more and more beautiful.

'I met **Princess Diana** through *Vogue*, with Anna Harvey and photographer Patrick Demarchelier, on the famous shoot that changed the way the world saw her. They didn't tell us she was going to turn up – she just arrived, and disarmed us immediately with her honesty and vulnerability.

'She wasn't a model, and she had never wanted to be regarded that way, so sometimes it would take a bit of persuading to get her used to a less structured way of doing her hair. She had her own style, and wanted to look slightly groomed. The "just-got-out-of-bed" look was never for her. She used to say to me, "Well, people are expecting Princess Diana, so I'd better not disappoint them." Towards the end of her life, she was more relaxed about these things – when she slicked back her hair, it was as if she was saying, "I don't need to hide behind my fringe, I'm happy to face the world." I encouraged her to go to Angola without a hairdresser. She had a big, thick mop of hair which was quite difficult to tame. If you're in the public eye your hair is harder to do than your make-up and you need a bit of moral support. Working with her was fun. I miss her like mad.

'As for the present day, **Gisele** arrived from Brazil and really put her stamp on the beginning of this century, and to me, she brings it all full circle. I met her on a Ralph Lauren shoot with Bruce Webber. Nicola Clarke bleached the ends of her hair white, and suddenly she looked a bit like a surfer albeit a very glamorous one. She has it all: Cindy Crawford, Linda Evangelista, Kate Moss, there is a bit of all of them in her, even in the way she poses.

'What has changed in the last 25 years? A lot of rules have been broken. People don't want to be dictated to. I try to make people feel gorgeous, sexy, healthy, well groomed. Nice shiny hair is sexy. Hair that looks as if you could touch it or run your hands through it, is sexy. You have to learn to love your hair. Even me, and I haven't got any.'

Why are most famous hairdressers men?

From Vidal Sassoon and John Frieda to Nicky Clarke, most of the famous hairdressers are male. It has been suggested that this is because beauty editors are mostly female and therefore like writing about the opposite sex, but I have to refute this. Otherwise all famous dermatologists, make-up artists, therapists, masseurs, etc., would also be men. The answer is, I don't know, and, disappointingly, none of the male hairdressers I asked would admit to knowing either.

LAURA PATTEN'S BLOW-DRY

Whenever the Deputy Beauty Editor at *Tatler* announces she's off to the hair-dressers in her lunch break, I groan with anticipation. How long will it take?

But back she comes, within an hour, with shiny, happy hair and the perfect straight blow-dry. Responsible for it is Jade at Michaeljohn, and this is how she does it:

'It's very simple. First you have to shampoo correctly, using a good conditioner, and remove the tangles while the hair is still wet. There's nothing worse than combing through tangles while drying, it really slows down the process. Then I apply a serum to help keep frizzy ends smooth. You put a few drops on the palm of your hand first, then rub down the mid-lengths and ends of your hair while it's still wet. Next you need the right hairbrush – we use a wooden-handled brush with a metal base and tough, inflexible plastic bristles. It's the metal base that is the important bit, as it retains the heat from the hairdryer as you pass the brush through the hair. A powerful hairdryer and strong arms are also important. You put the brush underneath each section of the hair, and run the hairdryer over the brush, keeping it close to the brush all the way down the length of the hair. There is no need to spend hours doing it. And we still have time for a good chat.'

HAIROLOGY: WHAT DOES IT ALL MEAN?

Like estate agents, hairdressers have their own language. Here's what some of the most commonly used terms actually mean:

Blunt/club: A way of cutting a straight line on a really sharp bob.

Graduation: Layering the edges of a haircut so that instead of it falling to one length, there is a curved line at the bottom. Graduated cuts are usually found on short to medium-length hair.

Movement: As in, 'Ooh, lots of lovely movement!', it means there is layering and texture in the style, but with softer, longer layers around the face.

Razor cutting: Cutting the hair with a special implement that results in a soft, broken-up, textured haircut. It takes a lot of weight away from the hair to make it look finer.

Slide cutting: This is the technique where you slide scissors through the hair for a wispy, feathery texture.

Texture: A loose term, used to describe choppy layers, so the overall effect is not smooth, flat or one length, but more ruffled. Meg Ryan would be the perfect example of someone whose hair has lots of 'texture'.

Finally, is it naff, or ultra-cool to call a hairdresser a hairdresser?

'I think it's a little old-fashioned, but it's not an insult,' says Worthington. 'I prefer "stylist". And we definitely say "apprentice" instead of "junior" for our trainees.' From the front-line of hairdressing, Peter Gray, a session stylist (that means he does catwalk shows and shoots but you won't ever get him to touch so much as a strand of your hair), has a reassuringly down-to-earth approach: 'It's okay to say hairdresser again,' he says. Phew.

TOP STYLES IN TEN MINUTES, NO 2: BIG HAIR PART ONE

Big, bouffy, sexy hair depends on the length of your hair. You're aiming for fullness, with chunkiness at the roots. Blow-dry roughly using a volumising product, a firm-hold gel or hairspray. If you have mid-length hair, crimp the roots underneath for the first two inches to give the hair fullness at the base. Don't crimp the top section of the hair – you'll need this to disguise the crimping underneath. On shorter hair you will have to resort to back-combing. Apply a putty-like product through the ends of the hair for guts and texture.

BIG HAIR PART TWO: IN TWO MINUTES

Hang your head upside down, tease the roots a little, spray and then go. It gives you volume in a dishevelled way.

HOW ANNOYING ARE YOU? WHAT BUGS HAIRDRESSERS THE MOST?

- 'Clients chatting on mobile phones when you're trying to do their hair.'
- Flipping magazines – 'We should really get easels, otherwise their heads keep moving from side to side.'
- 'Clients who fall asleep when you're doing their highlights – their heads nod forwards so it's impossible to put the foils in properly.'

You've been warned.

TOP STYLES IN TEN MINUTES, NO 3: THE MODERN CHIGNON

Worthington says the key to the perfect modern chignon is 'grabability'. 'It shouldn't look too contrived.' With this in mind, either work with hair that hasn't been freshly washed, or apply a light styling gel to the hair first to make it feel a little 'older'. This texture also helps the pins to stay in place. Smooth your hair into a ponytail at the back and then pin the tail randomly in a twist to the head.

TO TIP OR NOT TO TIP?

The golden rule is that if you feel you have had good service, you should be generous. You should consider tipping anyone who's been pleasant and looked after you well, from the apprentice up. The easiest way to give it to them is to leave it with the receptionist and either be specific as to who gets it or ask the receptionist to sort it out for you.

What is the biggest thing we get wrong?

Once a year, the Irish-born John Barrett flies over from New York for a charity marathon of hair-cutting and colouring at the Mandarin Oriental Hotel in London in aid of the Rehabilitation for Addicted Prisoners Trust (RAPT). He is a fantastic hair-cutter, who is legendary amongst New York society – he creates the kind of styles that look fabulous without leaving you looking like you just had your hair cut – all awkward and self-conscious and lacquered to within an inch of your life.

'It's not what a client does wrong, so much as what hairdressers do wrong,' he says. 'A woman will walk in and I can see from 100 yards what is wrong with her hair. Hairdressers don't look enough at a woman's skin tone. They forget that a haircut is not just a cut, it's a whole experience, and everything needs to be adjusted accordingly, whether it's the lipstick or a new pair of glasses. If, as a hairdresser, you've just given a haircut, then it's not enough – if the person needs it, you should also give advice. Everybody has one amazing feature, be it their eyes or their cheek-bones, or, if they're Julia Roberts or Cameron Diaz, then everything. We pick on that one amazing feature and focus on it.'

Say I can't wait for his once-yearly visits, and New York is out of bounds for a few months, how can I get that great haircut? 'The best way is to find someone who you see with a great hairstyle, whether it's someone you know already or a stranger on the street, and ask them who cuts it and where. When you're at that salon, if the hairdresser doesn't give you a consultation first or if they make you feel uncom-fortable, just get up and go.'

Cut is nothing without its partner in crime: colour. The days of having to pretend to be a 'natural' blonde, brunette or redhead are long since gone, thankfully, and now, there are no Brownie points to be earned by having mousy hair, even if it does mean you're a hair-colour virgin. In a good salon, you'll sit down with both the colourist and the cutter before anyone so much as even washes your hair. Both should discuss your style together – after all, there's not much point in having an elaborate head of highlights if what you're after is a classic Mary Quant bob. Or getting a flat vegetable semi-permanent colour to enhance the texture of your short, choppy 'Lulu' cut – it just won't work.

At Daniel Galvin's salon in Marylebone, London, rows and rows of women sit with silver foil wraps in their hair. They reckon they get through about three tons of foil a year. Hair salons are not glamorous places – thumbed copies of *Hello!*, empty coffee cups and mobile phones are the boring remains of their bored owners. Getting your hair done can take a long time. It's hard to believe that Madonna, Nicole Kidman and the late Princess Diana have all sat amongst the same remains, waiting for Galvin's magic hands to transform their mousy brown locks into something worthy of a paparazzi camera flash, but sat here they have, on full view for the general hair-colouring public, like those same copies of *Hello!* brought to life.

Galvin has been colouring hair for forty-two years and has also worked as the colour consultant for Wella and L'Oréal. One of the reasons he gets it right and makes the wait worthwhile is that he insists on a thorough consultation with all involved before he starts. The day I visited (short brown hair with grey strands sprouting everywhere) he actually cut a section of the entire length, from underneath the top layers where it wouldn't show, so that he could analyse what previous colourists had done. This is important because of any chemical reactions between differing products, particularly as often what the client is told is going on their hair may have a misleading name. 'Vegetable' colour, for example, is often semi-permanent colour, with peroxide in it, which is permanent and will penetrate the cortex, or second layer, of the hair. It can result in regrowth, i.e. when the hair grows the roots that come through will be the original, natural colour of the hair, with a sharp line dividing them from the dyed hair. Henna is the only completely natural vegetable colour and this isn't often used in salons because the results can be inconsistent and unpredictable. What the cutting taken from my hair shows is that there are dark and light bits of uneven colour where my hair has been dyed before, and then exposed to the sun. Galvin applies a pure vitamin C lotion mixed with water to the cutting to strip the hair of any colour still left behind. (He has patented this technique, incidentally, in a milder version to 'clean' the hair of any chemicals left behind and leave it in amazing condition.) From this, he can tell exactly how much of which type of hair colourant to apply, and get a more finely tuned result.

Apart from knowing what has been applied to the hair most recently the next most important discussion to take place between colourist and client is what colour or colours will suit the client best. Galvin is a firm believer in enhancing what you already have, in the same way that well-applied make-up will bring out the colour of your eyes or emphasise cheekbones. He even manages to be positive about my grey hairs, believing that grey hairs appear in order to soften the overall colour of the hair in sympathy with the appearance of the first lines on the face. My finished result, incidentally, is lots of blonde highlights over my natural brunette base, thus disguising the grey strands, without actually blanket-colouring brown all over them – it's very clever. 'Everyday colour,' he argues, 'shouldn't be too fashionable. People aren't scared of colour any more and will happily take an idea from the catwalk. But it has to suit the natural pigmentation of the hair, the complexion and the colour of the eyes.' He places a great deal of emphasis on the latter. 'We did Diana's colour for the last seven years or so of her life,' he says of his most famous blonde. 'Her natural hair colour was quite dark, and it was only by making it blonder that you could see how beautiful her eyes were.' (It's no coincidence that around 65 per cent of his female customers now go for blonde highlights.)

Galvin will spend around forty-five minutes discussing colour options with a client and doing strand and patch tests to ensure she is happy before embarking on a major change. Because often, however much a client thinks she wants a certain colour, it may not be what she really wants. 'You have to be a psychologist to an extent, and try to understand what people are thinking. Sometimes they'll say, "I want to be lighter," when what they really mean is, "I want to be brighter." The biggest kick I get is when a client comes out with a smile on her face and says, "I love it!"'

COLOURING AT HOME

Joanna Lumley once told me that she colours her own hair because she can't be bothered to wait for so long in hair salons. As she has beautifully thick-looking blonde hair, she's a good advertisement for home hair colourants. The most important thing you can do when doing it yourself is to read the instructions. Twice. Do a strand test and do a patch test. Make sure the colour you have chosen will suit you – a good guide if you're going lighter is to stay within two to three shades lighter than your natural colour. If things go wrong, admit defeat and head for a professional to get the colour rectified. Try your local salon or call a helpline, such as Wella's Consumer Hair Advisory Team.

WILLIAM ON COLOUR MISTAKES

William is a big, burly New Yorker who works at the John Barrett salon. He is a charmer. He took one look at my grey roots and said in his big, burly New York accent, 'What is it with the grey? Is that a British thing?' He is always right. Unlike us clients it would seem.

'The biggest mistake a client makes is becoming a colour junkie – doing too much hair colouring. This is quite common in New York where everyone is so over-maintained. The problem is that the hair becomes weaker in its structure and the colour doesn't hold, no matter what the colourist does. Ideally, you should try and get your highlights done every ten to twelve weeks. Another mistake is to see too many different colourists. They will all have different ideas and it's hard to achieve any kind of consistency. It also makes it harder for your current colourist to get an accurate picture of what was used on the hair before, although you will always have a ballpark picture. Wanting colour duplicated from a picture in a magazine never works – you'd be amazed at how many women will even show me black and white pictures and expect me to be able to recreate that colour! Pictures of Jennifer Aniston, J-Lo and Sophie Dahl are the ones we get most often. I would say impatience was the worst part of my job – the impatience of a client who wants you to get from dark brown to the palest of blondes in just one sitting, when they've already seen twenty different colourists. These are tint brushes, not magic wands!

'But the best thing about my work is the incredible people I meet, and the creative freedom they give me. It's amazing what people share with you. I consider this my second education.'

HAIROLOGY: WHAT DOES IT ALL MEAN?

Permanent colour: This type of colour will grow out, leaving the original root colour showing, but the advantage is you can colour your hair lighter as well as darker. A salon visit every six to eight weeks is usually required to retouch your roots.

Rinse/vegetable colour: This will only temporarily coat the hair shaft, and does not permanently colour the hair. It should wash out within six to eight washes. It also adds a glossy shine to dull and lifeless hair.

Semi-permanent: This lasts longer than a rinse or vegetable colour, but still only for a relatively short time, e.g. six to eight washes.

YOU HATE SPENDING TIME IN A SALON . . .

So make sure the colour you opt for is low maintenance. A semi-permanent or vegetable colour is best for low-maintenance hair, because either one will wash out leaving no long-lasting effects.

But as much in love with the whole process of colouring hair as Galvin is, like most hairdressers, he thinks condition is an intrinsically important aspect of having a good hairstyle, if not the most important. I remember growing up as the third long-haired girl in our family, with my mother religiously brushing my hair and plaiting it every day and every night (yes, we slept in plaits) for the first ten years or so of my life. She believed that keeping it tidy and out of the way would prevent it from knotting and tangling so easily, and therefore result in it looking in better condition. (Also I suspect that with five children in all it was easier for her to look after that way.) Being part-Burmese probably also had something to do with having healthy-looking hair – Asian hair does tend to look stronger – but one thing that certainly can't be afforded any credit was what she washed our hair with. Most of our shampoos came with 'ECONOMY' branding stamped all over them. Like most consumers then, she suspected there wasn't much one could really do to improve the condition of hair, short of slathering on conditioner to the ends, as hair is essentially, dead.

Well, yes and no. Hair is dead, but as an organic substance it is also incredibly strong and elastic, and the things you put on it, the elements you expose it to and the things you eat all go some way towards improving or harming its condition. What is it exactly? Think of a three-layered rope – compact, twisted, but very strong. The outer strand, known as the cuticle, is made up of interlocking scales, the second strand is the cortex, where the protein, melanin, the moisture and sulphur and salt bonds live. It's these that hold the hair together and form its shape. The third layer is the medulla, which has no known use, and isn't even apparent in some very fine hair. The interlocking scales on the outside allow things like shampoo, heat and chlorine to enter the cuticle. The problem with this is twofold – because the balance is so delicate, the scales can open too much, and let protein, an important component in maintaining hair strength, out. However, they can't open wide enough to allow certain, larger molecules such as the kind found in cheaper brands of shampoo – to enter.

It is therefore vital to choose the right products to look after your hair. One expert told me that if you take a section of your hair, near the front and gently scratch the scalp with your fingernail, in 90 per cent of cases you will find a white, flaky residue – the old shampoo and styling products you haven't washed away over time. The lower the quality of the products you use, the worse the residue will be, blocking the scalp and asphyxiating the hair follicle. The hair eventually becomes finer and finer, leading to breakages and a thinner head of hair overall. Think of it as depriving a plant of water and nutrition for a long period of time. It can hang on in there for a while, but eventually it will die.

But with so many shampoos to choose from, how do you find one that is right for you? The last time I looked at the shelf in Boots there was an over-whelming array of haircare products to choose from – around eighty different brands, each with its range of shampoos, conditioners, styling and colouring products. Who has the time to read every single label? It used to be the case that hair companies offered you a choice of three 'types', one of which your hair was supposed to correspond to: normal, greasy or dry. Much as in the skin-care market, labelling has improved, along with technology, with the result that if your hair is processed but long, oily at the scalp and dry at the ends, and you'd like a colour-enhancing brunette tinge to boot, the chances are there's a shampoo out there that claims to do it all. But there's still no simple way of finding a product to suit you, other than through sheer trial and error.

Trichologist Philip Kingsley, whose clients include Mick Jagger and Kate Winslet – both of whom have rather nice heads of hair – believes in the regime approach. I once chopped my hair off because I was so fed up with the main-tenance involved – one hair expert had put me on a routine that was so complicated I actually found myself sticking up a calendar in the shower and ticking off each wash. But routines are the way to go if you're serious about your hair.

'Women expect too much from a shampoo, when really they need a regime,' Kingsley argues. 'Washing your hair with shampoo will only cleanse it. The hair should be treated like the face, which we cleanse, tone, moisturise and then apply make-up to. You always need a shampoo. You always need a conditioner. You may need something for the scalp. You will need something to style it.'

To choose a range that suits you he advises either seeing someone like him or your own hairdresser, who can look at your scalp and advise you accordingly, or spending time to read the labels, being aware of certain chemical ingredients if you're allergic to something in particular and then trying the regime. He believes in using a good-quality shampoo from a range that invests in research and development, uses high-quality ingredients and gets the explanations on the bottles right – something which sounds simple enough but which in practice even larger companies can get wrong sometimes. And remember, it's only a shampoo. If you really want the all-singing, all-dancing, shiny, bouncy locks promised on the label, it's a good idea to look at your lifestyle. Still blow-drying your already-dry hair? Using heated irons? Cheap mousses? Eating badly? Smoking twenty a day? To my knowledge there's no shampoo that can deal with all these things just yet.

So, you've got your shampoo, conditioner, scalp treatment, fine ends serum, and goodness knows what else. Now what? The way you use the products is the next part of the battle. Here's how my hairwash goes. Get in bath. Wallow in one of the many free, totally delicious, pampering products I am sent. Read a magazine, getting the corners wet. Realise I have fifteen minutes before I have to run for the bus, and I'm too late to order a taxi as back-up. Dunk head in sudsy water. Tip a palmful of my baby's shampoo into my hand, and work it into a lather through my hair. Grab the shower attachment and rinse – Ow! Too hot! Aah! Too cold! Rub a palm-full of expensive conditioner into the ends of the hair, wiping the palm of my hand over the rest of it for good measure. Do not leave on for fiften minutes as instructed by label. Rinse with the shower attachment – Ow! Too hot! Aah! Too cold! Leap out of bath, wrap in towel, run a comb through hair, get dressed, and 'blow-dry' using the heating of the taxi I luckily manage to book over the phone. And then I wonder why my shampoo doesn't work.

Here's how it's supposed to go. Get in the bath or shower. Before wetting the hair, run a wide-toothed comb through the hair to remove any tangles. Grab the shower attachment and wet the hair with warm water – not too hot, not too cold. Make sure the underside of the hair is wet by running your fingers through your hair as the water pours over it. Pour a small amount (the proverbial 'walnut' size) of the shampoo you have spent days – if not weeks – selecting into the palm of the hand, rub your hands together, and then smooth it over your head. Aim for gentle massage movements rather than vigorous scratching, using your fingertips to gently knead the scalp. Do this for three minutes or so, running your fingers through the hair lengths from time to time, front to back to prevent tangles occurring. With the shower attachment, rinse with warm water, for longer than you think is necessary – apparently none of us rinses for long enough. Pour a small amount of conditioner into the palm of your hand, rub palms together and apply to the ends, smoothing over the mid-lengths, but avoiding the scalp. Rinse straight away or leave for as long as the manufacturer recommends. Rinse again, then wrap in a towel to absorb excess moisture, and comb with that wide-toothed comb. But you knew all that really, didn't you?

Leave-in conditioners are also excellent for leaving out a final stage of the rinsing process, if time really is of the essence. They weren't really designed to be time-saving, but as a way of protecting the hair for longer. I've long been a fan of Phyto 7, a plant-based cream with rosemary, sage and bay to detangle and strengthen the hair from Phytologie, a French company, so I was a little concerned to hear that apparently all leave-in conditioners are bad for the hair as they just collect dust. Lee Bradley from Phytologie assures me that this is only the case with ones that are made with a high silicone content, and even though I know he is paid to defend his corner, I do believe him, as it's one of the best conditioners I know. He also says that if you're using a wash-out conditioner, keep rinsing until the hair no longer feels 'soggy' with the stuff. If you don't wash it out properly it can have the opposite effect, and your ends when dry will feel brittle. And the only cure for split ends, as we know, is to cut them off.

How can you find a good trichologist?

For some reason – perhaps because at the end of the day we all want to believe in miracles – when it comes to hair there are some real cowboys out there who promise the earth, don't deliver, but still charge a fortune. Think of your trichologist as being like a dentist for the hair. He or she should be able to advise on the best way to care for your hair, recommending products, and telling you how to handle your hair, e.g. if it is streaked how to stop it from breaking. Your trichologist should be able to achieve an improved cosmetic appearance and look after the hair in the long term, perhaps by offering blood tests. Contact the Institute of Trichologists and ask for a registered qualified member who is independent of any commercial company.

What if your conditioner makes your hair look finer?

If you find your hair is naturally fine and seems even finer after conditioning, you are probably either using the wrong product for your hair type or are not rinsing thoroughly enough.

What about the build-up myth?

There used to be a brand of shampoo whose whole raison d'être was to 'prevent build-up'. You had to change your shampoo every so often, it argued, because your hair got used to the same brand, and the shampoo would build up and refuse to be rinsed away. Lee Bradley argues that there is such a thing as build-up, but that it doesn't just affect the hair but the scalp as well. 'The hair looks dull and feels like nylon,' he says. 'It's not so much your shampoo that is at fault, more the fact that when you bought the shampoo you bought it to treat a specific condition. It's a snapshot of the way your life was then.' If that condition no longer exists, e.g. an oily scalp, you should move on to another shampoo. 'If you keep overdoing the treatment on any aspect of your haircare it won't work any more.' You need to take a good look at your haircare routine every eight to twelve weeks.

How often should you wash your hair?

Some hair experts recommend washing your hair daily to ensure a healthy-looking shine. I have always thought this too much and too boring, especially when I had really long hair, but perhaps if I'd combed it through first it wouldn't have been so tedious.

I am relieved to hear that there is another school of thought that suggests washing hair every two or three days should be enough. The reason is that daily washing will remove the hydrolypidic film (a mixture of urea, sweat and sebum on the hair's surface), which is a device that Nature invented to prevent our bodies from being attacked by bacteria and fungus, and to provide us with the moisture needed to prevent our skin and scalp from becoming dehydrated. Frequent washing with a detergent-based shampoo removes the film for eight to nine hours a day, leaving us more open to intolerances to day-to-day products as well as to fungal and bacterial infections. That's one reason why haircare companies are reporting a massive upturn in hair sensitivity – we all need to be a bit dirtier. Either way, to my brother Rupert Baird-Murray, if you're reading this (unlikely, I admit) and all those male soap-shirkers out there who insist that a quick dunk in your bath-water is all you need: it's not. Once a week would be a start.

Why if you're black you need to be rich when it comes to hair

At least, that's what Ateh Damachi, the beauty assistant at Tatler says. 'I worked out once that it would cost me £175 a month to maintain my hair.' She has a short slick bob. How does she reach that figure? 'If you want healthy, glossy hair, you need two deep conditioning treatments in a salon once a month, and you'll also need to get your hair relaxed every six to eight weeks.' There are some things you can do yourself – Ateh applies a deep conditioning treatment each week, wraps her hair in cling film, and then wraps a towel around it before watching the omnibus edition of EastEnders. 'That's how I know when the job's done! You have to condition often, because the process of relaxing your hair makes it very porous, and it's not good to wash it too often, not more than once or twice a week.'

She will never, ever attempt to relax her hair herself. 'I once asked a hairdresser why she became a hairdresser and she said it was because she had gone to someone who had burnt all her hair off so that she was forced to wear a wig for six months. She swore that from that day on no one would ever lay a finger on her hair, and went to beauty school. It's an extreme case, but I am always hearing horror stories, and I would strongly recommend you use a professional.'

The future for Afro hair is positive. 'I do think there will be a real surge in pro-ducts for mixed race hair,' says Ateh. 'Not least because mixed couples are having *babies and the mums haven't a clue how to cope with their children's hair! I'll just be glad when I don't have to hike to Kilburn or Hackney or Brixton on a monthly raid for black hair products and can buy them in Boots like everyone else.'*

What's so good about pure plant ingredients?

Products made with pure plant oils are more likely to be absorbed by the hair than those made from chemical or synthetic ingredients, because the plant molecules are closer in shape and size to our own hair molecules. Chemicals are perfect spheres, whereas the molecules that make up our bodies, hair and scalp are imperfect, irregular shapes.

Of course, there are worse problems than lank locks. About 65 per cent of Kingsley's female clients come to see him because of hair loss, a condition about which there has been a fair bit of scaremongering lately, with the media claiming it is on the rise amongst women. Whatever the statistics, or alleged statistics, its effect on the female psyche is devastating. We're not supposed to lose our hair, right? Men lose their hair, not women. One twenty-three-year old girl went to see Kingsley in a bad state because her hair was falling out. Her family hair history – the fact that most of the women in her family also had thinning hair – pointed to a genetic tendency for her to suffer the same problem. Compounding it all was the fact that she had called a telephone support group who had 'helpfully' advised her to just accept it and stop worrying about it as, after all, her mother had the same hair type. Her family doctor had told her that if it got really bad she could always wear a wig. With friends like these . . . In fact, the special haircare programme she had been put on by Kingsley had started to work, but, as he'll be the first to admit, these things take time, and when you're confronted with an image in the mirror of a thinning head of hair every day, it's hard to remain positive. The psychological effect on his client proved to be so traumatic that she not only blamed her mother for everything, but refused to leave the house for a while.

It's not surprising there is no instant solution, contrary to what many charlatans of the industry would have you believe. First, the type of hair loss varies. What most of us refer to as hair loss is in fact reduction in hair volume. The actual diameter of the hair looks thinner and the overall effect is one of loss of hair body. Hair loss can also be a receding hairline or, more rarely, patches appearing on the crown. Second, you have to establish what the conditions are that led to the hair loss in the first place – stress, hormonal problems, certain HRT drugs, bad diet, incorrect haircare. It takes a while to assess how each is affecting the client. In some cases, it may be appropriate to ask for a blood test, which may show if you have enough iron and other vital minerals for your hair. Kingsley says, 'I ask a lot of pertinent questions about what my clients eat, and also when they eat. If they're of reproductive age, sometimes the iron levels may be too low.' Third, you need to be patient. It took about three to five years for that hair to get there in the first place. Now you've lost it, it's not going to grow back overnight.

Another kind of hair loss that affects women, albeit temporarily, is post-partum hair loss. My husband was almost driven mad by the long strands of brown hair – mine – that appeared throughout the house on almost every surface in the months that followed the birth of our son. No one seems to know why hair loss after birth happens, although at a guess I'd say it's surprising your arms, legs and head don't fall off as well when you consider the general trauma your body goes through in the whole pregnancy and birth experience. Kingsley once did a study at the Cuckfield Maternity Hospital over a period of three years to try and establish why some women lost their hair after childbirth and not others. He found no correlation with diet or sexual activity, or any of the other factors one might assume could contribute to it. All he found was that 50 per cent of women did lose their hair and 50 per cent didn't, and that women with multiple pregnancies had thinner hair than those with just one child or two. The other thing he found was that what happens first time round in childbirth bears no relation to what happens the second or third time around. What did I do about my own hair? I cut it short, at which point my husband said, 'Why have you cut your hair? It looked so much nicer longer.'

Just as unsexy as hair loss is that other problem: dandruff. What can I say about dandruff to make it more interesting? A friend of mine – now a reformed character, you'll be glad to hear – used to refer to cocaine as 'the devil's dandruff'. This is possibly a little too politically incorrect for a beauty book, so let's move on quickly to the other interesting thing I've come across about dandruff. For some reason there are rather a lot of home remedies in existence. This is either because their creators assume that if you have great big flecks of white on your shoulders you won't be going out much, and therefore will have time to concoct a few lotions and potions at home, or more likely, it's because natural remedies, essential oils and mild chemicals are a more attractive way to clear up the problem than the sometimes foul-smelling, rather powerful anti-dandruff shampoos on the market. (They *do* work, incidentally, but what you should probably do is try to alternate them with your usual shampoo and avoid anything that leaves your hair looking dull or excessively greasy – again, it's a question of trial and error.)

What most home remedies have in common is the ability to cleanse the scalp of any build-up of dead skin cells. This occurs when the normal bacteria that live on the skin, such as sebum, go into overdrive as a result of changes to our metabolic rate, increased stress, hormonal changes, or a sudden shift in diet to include too much sugar, salt or fat. When the sebum pushes through the hair follicles, it is absorbed by the dead skin cells. It then sticks together and clings to the scalp, giving the appearance of even larger white flakes. It's really not attractive.

Try Sue Brandon's concoction from *The Complete Handbook of Beauty Tips* of rosemary, thyme, lavender, or juniper, in the form of an infusion or essential oils. Massaged into the scalp after shampooing, it has cleansing and antiseptic properties. She also suggests boiling half an ounce of sage leaves in 1 litre of water for five minutes, allowing it to cool, and then massaging it into the scalp; or to make it easier to wash away the flakes, try dissolving an aspirin in your shampoo. Philip Kingsley's cure is to continue with your favourite shampoo (and let's face it, if it takes as long as I think it does to find the perfect one, you might not want to give it up so quickly), apply your regular conditioner to the ends, rinse well, dry gently with a towel and, before styling, sprinkle your scalp with an anti-flaking tonic. If the only tonic you've used before is the one that goes with gin, try his tonic recipe, made from equal quantities of witch hazel and mouthwash.

If it gets really bad, it's time to hand the mixing over to your local chemist. Kingsley suggests you ask them to make you up an oil-in-water emulsion containing 1 per cent sulphur and 1 per cent salicylic acid crystals. You apply the cream to your scalp in one-inch partings, massage it in for five to ten minutes, wrap your head in a warm, damp towel for a further five to ten minutes, and shampoo as normal, finishing with the scalp tonic, above. If your scalp feels at all irritated, or as if it is burning, wash it off straight away – you may be one of the very small percentage of people with an allergy to sulphur.

Finally, to have beautiful hair, be careful what you do to it. It sounds obvious, but all that blow-drying, curling, tonging and straightening does take its toll, as any model or actress will testify. I remember asking one stylist as I heard my hair hissing under a straightening iron and saw the steam rise, whether this was doing any harm to it. 'No, of course not. I put hairspray on it first to protect it.' Hmm . . . Another time I was rushed off the set of a commercial – ironically for hair – when someone had lowered the burning studio lights a little too close in order to maximise the shine on my hair for the benefit of the cameras. I could actuallly smell burning, and apparently steam was seen to rise from my head. The truth is, that when it comes to getting what they want for a picture, some hairdressers just don't care.

DOS AND DON'TS TO PREVENT HAIR LOSS

Do eat lots of oily fish and green vegetables such as Savoy cabbage.
Do eat regularly and evenly – rather than having one main meal a day, eat several at evenly spaced intervals, and take your time to eat each meal properly.
Do rinse your hair properly after washing it, for at least two minutes.

Don't smoke or drink too much alcohol – it affects women's hair more than men's. Drinking can build up testosterone levels in the scalp and trigger the signal for the hair follicle to die.

DOS AND DON'TS ON HOLIDAY

You'll be bringing less back with you, unless you look after it in the sun. Even if you have the most perfect head of hair before you go, fourteen days in the sun will rip the life out of it. It's the equivalent to blasting your hair with a hairdryer for eight hours every day. Chlorine and salt water will dry it out even more.

Do use a protective hair product that will deflect UVA and UVB rays. Or wear a hat or scarf.

Do tell your colourist you're going away if you're getting highlights done – sophisticated tones of platinum will lose their subtlety, while other blonde lights will take on a more intense, sunkissed look.

Do use a shampoo that can remove salt water and chlorine, and wash daily.

Do use an after-sun or intensive conditioner for the hair, in the same way as you would for your skin.

Do change your regular shampoo and conditioner when you return. You'll need something to put the moisture back.

Don't think that putting olive oil in your hair, or leaving your regular conditioner in all day as a 'mask' will protect it. Conditioners contain plastics and fats, so all you're doing is frying your hair.

Don't bother colouring your hair darker before you go away. The sun will always take it down a notch or so, resulting in instant colour fade.

'Your feet's too big. No one likes you 'cos
your feet's too big . . .'
The Ink Spots

Chapter Five

THE OTHER HANDSOME FRENCHMAN

My father, my lovely father, used to say, 'Never trust a man who can dance.' This was really to make up for the fact that he hated dancing, and suffered the same chronic embarrassment as I did on the rare occasions when either of us had to do so in public. On my wedding day, we shuffled round the dance floor together so desperately self-conscious as not remotely to enjoy the moment, never mind seize the day. My grandmother used to say, jokingly, 'Who do you think is looking at you anyway?' and she was right. By the second bar of what-ever song it was, everyone was busily back at the champagne.

'Never trust . . .' is an expression that can just as easily be applied to people with good hands and feet. Never trust someone with beautifully manicured hands, or tenderly cared for feet, because what on earth are they doing with their lives? Where do they find the time? Why aren't they digging big holes or bashing out books on a computer, or ruffling the fur of small dogs or big men, or baking five-tier cakes, or cleaning the hooves of racehorses like the rest of us? Again, like my father, my suspicion stems from how I feel when I look at my own nails: chronically embarrassed. They are short, they are often dirty, and at least two or three of them sport different-coloured nail polishes – I am always trying out colours. One of them has a nasty ridge down it which just won't mend. And, horror of horrors, I have chewed several of them down to the flesh after they have torn and I haven't been able to lay my hands on an emery board. (Emery boards, incidentally, belong to the same Bermuda Triangle as Post-It notes, pens and hair elastics. They disappear from your desk within seconds.)

The only time you can trust someone with beautifully manicured hands is when they're a hand model. How else can anyone justify such care and attention unless they're making fistfuls of cash from it? It is one of those jobs people can't quite believe is actually a job.

One of the most famous hand models in the world is a sixty-five-year-old American woman called Linda Rose, who has, since retiring, developed her own line of hand and feet products, including one for the legs that is gloriously entitled 'Dance All Night'. (You see, there we go again, the dancing thing . . .) It all started in 1954, when she was sixteen, and working as a model while going to college. Her agency called and said, 'Can you write a movie star's name across a picture?' from which we can only presume the movie star either couldn't write or had hideous hands. From that point Rose, who could do both, was much in demand, making $70 a day, which was a fortune in those days, but it still wasn't properly recognised as a job. 'The ultimate put-down,' she recalls, 'was when people would introduce you, saying, "This is Linda Rose. She's a model but she just does hands." They were still saying that when I had fourteen commercials on air that also showed my face.'

Rose retired from hand modelling when she was fifty-five years old, by which time she had made over 5000 commercials and print advertisements. The reason she was so popular over other girls with beautiful hands was that she was very dexterous with her fingers. 'I frosted a cake with a paper knife; I got on with children and pets – many were pet food commercials. Once I even had a bird relieve himself on my hands for Dove soap.' It became a challenge. Being able to take everything in her stride also helped her popularity with directors. 'Your tension shows first in your hands,' she says. While her hands looked immaculate in front of the cameras, the rest of the time they were raising two children who were born only fifteen months apart. 'My agent said, "You won't have a career, you know, your hands are going to go." To which I'd reply, "Well, in that case, the good Lord will find something else for me to do."'

'Hands that don't do anything are not very sexy. If you don't use them, you lose them. I like to feel the earth in the garden. I had two kids. I wasn't going to be anything but hands on, and I just figured that I wasn't going to restrain myself because of my hands. Your hands are supposed to be useful, comforting instruments of love, and nothing should hamper that.'

When real life did get in the way it was never from doing the more rumbustious things one imagines will be 'dangerous' for the condition of hands, such as chopping onions, or gardening, but more from doing ordinary things like getting out of the car. 'But I don't use them as utensils either. You won't catch me scratching things off a kitchen cabinet.'

HAVING BEAUTIFUL HANDS WITHOUT SPECIALISED HAND PRODUCTS

Linda Rose: 'An easy way to revive tired-looking hands is to take a little salt and some Vaseline and gently exfoliate to remove the layer of dead skin. If you can spare a little of your expensive face cream, your pores will more readily receive it. Then sleep overnight with gloves on (the thin plastic kind you get with home hair colourants). But not every night, otherwise you'll have revived hands and a very disgruntled husband.'

HAND PRODUCTS TO AVOID

Anything that contains formaldehyde. 'In a base coat, formaldehyde will immediately strengthen your nails, but after a month or so it damages them,' says Rose.

EMERGENCY NAIL REPAIRS

If you have a crack, take some nail glue, apply it to the nail and close the crack. Wipe it with some nail polish remover so that the glue doesn't penetrate the nail bed, then take a piece of tissue and a base coat polish, or a top coat polish, dab the tissue with the polish and put it on over the break. Take a little nail polish remover and smooth it over, then repeat the process three times: base coat, then remover. Linda uses coffee filters instead of tissue paper, as she finds these the ideal thickness.

GARDENING OR BEAUTIFUL NAILS: WHAT'S IT TO BE?

You can have both. Rub your nails over a bar of soap before you garden so you protect the cuticle. Wash your hands after gardening to get rid of the dirt and the soap.

WAVING, NOT DROWNING

If you want to have a long soak in the bath for hours, keep your hands out. All that water causes the skin to shrivel and isn't great for the nails.

AGE SPOTS

When you get those brown marks on your hands, invest in a bleaching treatment specially designed for hands. Before you get them, use a hand cream with a sunscreen.

SOME OTHER 'HOUSEHOLD' REMEDIES

- Lemon juice gets rid of hard-to-remove dirt. Just rub a wedge over finger nails and hands.
- Oatmeal applied to moist hands works well as an alternative to soap – it exfoliates at the same time.
- Sugar is great for removing stains like ink or oil. Mix it in equal proportions with sesame or sunflower oil, then rub over the hands to softly exfoliate.

I don't suppose I will ever have hands like Linda Rose's, even if I stop that nasty habit of scratching things off kitchen cabinets. I once had a manicurist come to my desk once a week for six weeks (this is a purely legitimate exercise as a beauty editor, and it comes under research). She was a lovely woman, and nurtured my nails until they started to look as if they might think about growing strong and long. Even with her coming to see me, I didn't apply the oil I was supposed to apply, and about three weeks after she stopped (even research has its limitations) so did I. No more filing and whatever it was I had promised I'd do.

Marian Newman is a manicurist who has worked on shoots with photographers like Nick Knight and Mario Testino. If you see a beautifully turned out pair of hands in an ad, nine times out of ten, she filed and buffed and smoothed them into shape. She is great to work with. She has lots of gossip (boringly, without the names of those concerned – she is far too discreet for that) and always does your nails while you're hanging around. (I know, I know, it's a tough job.) She works under a lot of pressure. On shoots there is an unofficial hierarchy – actually, there's nothing unofficial at all about it – everyone knows their place, from the photographer and editor down to the lowliest of the low, the studio assistant (make that two sugars, please). Nail technicians, as manicurists are now known, aren't quite as lowly as the tea-makers, but they slot in right after hair and make-up, by which time no one has the patience to wait for long. Very often they'll bring an assistant, so they can do a hand each, but you can forget about waiting for the polish to dry.

Quite often, if acrylic nail extensions are called for, the nail technician will also get a fair bit of resistance from the models. You can't blame them. 'I think false nails are terrible,' says our Number One hand model, Linda Rose. 'When I was modelling, if I had to match a particular star's hands, I wouldn't want to say no, but it does such damage to your nail. I have letters from people saying they don't have the nerve to take off their acrylics – they worry about what they will look like underneath'

Newman puts it down to bad execution, and then bad removal when the time comes. 'Models can be really wary of letting me put on artificial nails because they think I will damage their own nails, but I don't. I put temporary nails on and take them off at the end of the shoot,' she says. 'You have to go to someone with the right experience, the right training and the right under-standing.' Your nails will not grow better with artificial nails on top, but if that's why you're doing it, what you should do is to keep moisturising your own nails while you have the artificial ones on top. Then, in two to three months' time, take off the artificial ones, and the new part of your nail will have grown stronger because you have been applying an oil moisturiser, while the old part of your nail will be in exactly the same condition. 'But the technician needs to educate the client,' adds Newman. 'It's no good just whacking on a set of artificial nails and saying, "Up you get!"' And the most important thing of all is once they're on, don't pick. Newman claims to be the world's worst culprit – she wears arti-ficial nails the whole time because she is always trying out new products.

Newman has created huge, spiral silver artificial nails for a Givenchy *haute couture* show, and will often create elaborate metallic airbrushed finishes, but her favourite nails are those which look healthy and natural. 'I like doing that more than anything,' she says. Apparently they're easy to achieve. This I can hardly believe, knowing how difficult I have found it, but she insists, 'You don't need to have a huge maintenance routine with nails. It boils down to three simple things done regularly.'

I am on tenterhooks.

'The most important thing of all is to massage oil or hand cream into the cuticle and around the nail. A nail oil is best, applied at least once a day, but if that's too much trouble . . .'

'Olive oil?' I offer.

'Olive oil is fine, or a vegetable cooking oil, or almond oil, which is very good. Whatever. Oils with mineral oils in, like liquid paraffin, are not particu-larly good because the molecules are too big to penetrate. They will soften, but they won't penetrate.'

'And I just massage it in. No technique, no pressure points, no . . .'

'Just rub it in! The second really, really important thing is to take the edge of the nail off every week with a very fine emery board. You get your hair trimmed every couple of months because the ends get split. Well, the ends of your nails get dry, and they need removing as well.'

'Filing too . . . okay.' (A quick file once in a while, providing I can find that emery board, can't be too difficult.)

'But you have to do it weekly. Nails are made up of several layers, and the layers start to fray, just like split ends. By filing weekly, you are removing the frayed bits and getting back to the original, healthy nail. If you use a very harsh emery board the layers will split, but if you use a very fine sandpaper board and just sand it, they will be smooth, and with no snags.'

'But if you're trying to grow your nails, won't that just make them shorter?'

'No, because you're not taking any off, all you're doing is smoothing the edge. And if you follow that with a three-way buffer, which is the next thing, you'll seal the edges, get a perfectly smooth nail, and protect it from water seeping inside. Once water seeps inside, the layers of the nail start coming apart and peeling.' (In case you missed a bit, you oil, you file and you buff. That is it. Isn't that great? You need never have horrible nails again. You can stop right here and never read another thing about nails, which, let's face it, are only marginally more interesting than hair removal in the greater scheme of things. So that was oil, file and buff. Got it?)

For those of you who are still interested, we shall now move on to advanced nails. This means polish, sooner or later. I'll leave colours down to the subtle differences between seasons and fashion statements, street style and whatever the nail bar is offering this week, i.e. that is for you to decide on. The rule is to apply a base coat, then two thin layers of your chosen colour, followed by a top coat. And it's fine for your nails – it may even protect them.

MARIAN NEWMAN'S PERFECT FRENCH MANICURE

This is one of the hardest things to do. Most people use the side of the brush and sweep the white opaque polish over the edge. In fact, the best way is to hold the brush flat to the nail, and paint the white line on the edge of the nails in several tiny strokes, taking it slowly and carefully round the edge, following what is technically known as the 'smile line', where the edge of the nail goes from pink to white. A perfect French manicure has absolutely sharp points right in the extreme corners. These points are technically known as 'dog's ears', because they look like the points on dogs' ears.

Start by painting over the whole nail with a clear pink or peach-toned polish. Next, with the white polish, paint in your dog's ears, concentrating on getting the points absolutely sharp. Join one dog's ear to the next, following the natural shape of the smile line. Finish with a top coat. I would recommend you use an actual top coat and not just a clear polish, as it tends to be harder and will be more resistant to knocking and chipping for longer.

MARIAN NEWMAN'S PERFECT RED NAILS

'The brush is the most important thing here, and this is really where you get what you pay for. The more expensive nail polishes tend to have good-quality brushes, whereas the cheaper brands have brushes that look like chimney sweeps'. A good-quality brush, if you press it down on a hard surface, will fan out to a perfect curve. That curve is usually the perfect shape for a cuticle. Apply a base coat first. With your red polish, lift the brush out and wipe it on the edge of the bottle away from you, so that the majority of the paint will end up on the side of the brush that will go down on to the nail first. Place the loaded brush on the centre of the nail, then take the brush to the cuticle, press it, and it should form a perfect curve. This way, you don't flood the cuticle with paint and make loads of mistakes, getting polish all over the skin and so on. You then draw the brush straight up the middle, and in this way, you have the main part of the nail finished, and you only have tiny side bits to do.

Some people say you should paint the nail in three strokes, but I don't agree with this – it depends on so many other things, like how thick your polish is.

But don't do too many strokes either, otherwise the polish will dry before you finish. You shouldn't need to dip the brush back in the pot again. If you get the polish on the skin, take an orange stick, dip it in nail polish remover, and wipe it around the skin, or use a corrector pen. Finish with a top coat, and reapply the top coat every two to three days.

SPECIAL EFFECTS: HOW TO SHOW OFF WITH NAIL POLISH

'This is really easy,' says Marian Newman. 'Apply a base colour, then put two blobs in one corner of the nail in whichever colours you like. They can be toning, contrasting, whatever. With a pin, swirl them together – you'd be amazed. The combinations I love are a very dark blue, with a white and a red swirled together – it looks like fireworks. Or subtle colours like pale pinks, with a deeper pink and a silvery glitter swirled together.'

How can I get my polish to dry more quickly?

Marian Newman says: 'Cold water is the only thing. Wait until your nails are touch dry – say five minutes – and then put them in iced water or run them under a cold tap.'

The cuticle obsession . . . is all about . . .

Boredom, I'm convinced. Pushing the skin back against the nail bed whiles away the time, and it has to be better than biting your nails. 'You don't push back,' says Newman. 'A lot of people are obsessed with trying to expose the whole thing, whereas what you should do is gently scrape back the skin where it is stuck to the nail plate. In my opinion, cuticle removing creams with AHAs are the best, because the cream by its nature is moisturising, and the AHAs are excellent at removing dead skin cells and encouraging cell renewal. But you can't just use it once and expect it to work – you have to use it regularly. If you massage your nails regularly with oil, that will stop the cuticle sticking to the nail because it only sticks to the nail in the first place because it is dry.'

Which lasts longer – cheap polish or expensive?

Neither. If anything, it's the way you apply the polish: two thin coats over a base coat and under a top coat. You don't have to wait for each coat to dry in between. Most special quick-drying formulas are more brittle and will chip off more easily because they don't move with the nail. If nail polish is allowed to dry slowly, it will be more flexible. If you buff your nails first to a high shine, and then put nail polish on, it will last for longer.

Which way do you file?

Think of a piece of plywood. If you imagine it cut in a curve like your nails are, there would be a rough edge and a smooth edge. If you go the wrong way, it's going to snag. Work side to middle; and then on the other side, side to middle. It's like stroking a cat.

How important is diet?

Unless you are ill, not many people suffer from a bad diet. A good diet is obviously going to help your skin, hair and nails, but it is not going to make that much differ-ence. Environment is more important – what you're doing with your nails on a daily basis.

How annoying are we?

In a nail bar, you are very annoying if you persist in biting your skin. 'Nail biting is one thing – it's not very nice but you can hide it,' says Newman. 'But if you touch the skin surrounding the nail you can tell straight away if someone has been biting it. It looks disgusting, it affects the new nail, and you can get bumpy nails from doing it.'

You are even more annoying if you won't wait for your polish to dry. 'Everyone knows that nail varnish takes ages to dry. If you've spent ages doing someone's nails and they won't wait, they will invariably smudge it, and then say, "Oh, look what I've done!"'

Can you mend a split nail?

A vertical split at the end of the nail will not be cured if you can see that it runs all the way down to the half-moon at the base. If there is what looks like a ridge in the base, as the new nail grows, because it is soft, it moulds itself over the ridge and grows up as a split.

Do nail hardeners work?

The important thing is to use the correct one for your nails and never over-use them. 'When I was in the salon,' says Newman, 'clients would say, "I bought this hardener and used it on my nails and it was fantastic, but two weeks later they all broke off." That's because hardeners are only designed to be used until your nails improve, and then your nails become brittle and will snap. Some people will need them for longer than others.'

Is there a product that will make nails grow longer more quickly?

Your nails are dead, but grow from the base. You can increase the rate of growth by massaging, but there is no specific product you can paint on that will actually stimulate growth.

What do you do if your nails are brittle?

If you have hard, brittle nails, you must never use a hardener, but instead use a moisturiser to make them more flexible. Don't use it for too long, otherwise you will end up with bendy nails.

How do you find a good nail bar?

Nail bars are springing up all over the place, but it doesn't mean they're any good. There is no legislation or governing body that regulates the hygiene and general standards of nail bars in this country. Newman says, 'A guideline is, when you walk in, what is the atmosphere like? Are the desks clean? Are the shelves clean? Doing nails generates a lot of dust but that's no excuse for not cleaning it up. What sort of nails does the manicurist have? How much experience has she? Ask a simple question, such as, 'What is it that makes my nails peel?' If the answer seems logical, then the chances are the person knows what they're talking about. If it's a lot of waffle, move on. They have probably had some product knowledge training, but the important thing is, why is this happening in the first place?'

Why do nails peel?

Not enough moisture in them. Apply creams, or oil.

When it comes to feet, Bastien Gonzales, a French podiatrist, calls nail polish Public Enemy Number One. He swears that painting nail polish on your toes is tantamount to putting a plastic coating on your skin – the nail cannot breathe. It may even encourage fungus to grow.

Personally, while it might look unattractive, there are certain stages of my childhood when allowing fungus to grow on one's toenails would have been a distinct advantage, raising one's social status at school, and providing the added interest factor of always having something to look at during those moments of boredom. It might even be something worth cultivating now. You could entertain small children for hours. You could develop a range of nail polish kits that would help you grow crops of mushrooms, a bit like those polystyrene mushroom farms everyone kept in their cellars in the Seventies next to their wine and beer kits. It's all very organic, and anti-GM, which is also all very now. But small children aside, I can see how fungus on your toes might not look so great in a pair of Manolos.

So in the great war of nail polish, who is right? Are we for it or against it?

'M'lud, nail polish on your toes is quite a different matter from that worn on your fingers. First there is the style factor. A classic Chanel red is all very well on toes, but looks quite brassy on long fingernails. Worn on short, square fingernails it can look ultra-fashionable, but only on those capable of not looking like barmaids.

'Objection, Your Honour. It doesn't take a fashion victim to tell that fashions date, and how can my learned friend predict that long fingernails painted in Chanel red won't be the big thing in hands next season?'

'Objection sustained. Continue.'

'Moreover, M'lud, with regard to the question of fungus, one presumes that one's hands, when painted with polish of whichever colour [looks with mock deference to adversary] are not covered with socks and shoes all day, are they? One's hands, in other words, receive the benefit of our fresh, albeit somewhat polluted, air in continuous circulation around one's painted fingers? Therefore, one concludes, it is this difference in environment, coupled with the painting of one's toes, that contributes to a possible increase in the chances of obtaining said fungus. And that one would have to keep the polish on for a very long time indeed before such conditions might occur . . .'

Life is too short. Can you see how ridiculous this debate is becoming? The long and the short and the square-filed and the oval-filed of it all is take your polish off regularly, and if you're a polish addict, give your nails the odd chance to 'breathe'. Some people are naturally prone to fungal infections, or a minor cut near the nail, or over-zealous pushing back of the cuticles can trigger something nasty, in which case get some professional help.

Back to the lovely Bastien. I have a hard time describing Bastien. He is, in his own words, a 'pedicurist' but he trained as a 'podologue'. What this means is that he has all the skills of a chiropodist and pedicurist, i.e. he can make your feet look beautiful, but he also has the knowledge of a podiatrist – he knows about the intricate workings of our feet. He won't apply nail polish, but after one of his pedicures you won't need it; the toenails are left as delicately pink as the inside of a conch shell on a Caribbean beach. He buffs them to a smooth shine with diamond-coated dentist drills, finishing with a chamois leather. He trims away the dead skin on your feet and massages your calves with lavender and rosemary oils. He is very charming, and it's not surprising that he is flown all over the world, besides his usual bases of London and Paris, to treat his clients' feet. Why does this handsome young Frenchman want to spend his days bent double over men's and women's feet?

'It's strange how I got into this,' he says. 'I was a ski instructor and I tore a ligament. I went to see the doctors in Paris and they told me to stop. I stayed in Paris for six months, recovering from the operation, and after one month I was completely bored. I had a friend who made orthopaedic platforms for shoes and I became fascinated by the way you could restore the equilibrium of the foot . . .' (No, I'm not getting it. I am clearly going to have to start adding some exclamation marks so you get some idea of just how excited this man gets by feet.) 'I fell in love with pedicures! It was so interesting! Did you know that 85 per cent of ingrowing toenails can be cured just by a good pedicure? Pointy shoes and high heels can result in bad corns, but they can be cured in seconds!' he enthuses. 'People can walk like new people, and I love that!'

After studying podiatry, he worked in Burgundy before returning to Paris. On a trip back home to Bordeaux for his great grandmother's ninety-second birthday he was struck by how diligently she would buff her nails and how beautifully shiny they looked, even though she never applied polish.

He returned to Paris determined to recreate this natural shine on toenails. The problem was he could get the shine, but if a client had ridges in their toenails, the shiny nail still didn't look beautiful naturally. Fortunately, a holiday job plastering walls he had once had while still a student gave him the inspiration he needed. 'I found four different surfacing tools, like the ones we had used plastering, and made a cream with marble dust in it – when you apply the chamois leather over the cream it makes the nails go really shiny.'

The tools he talks about are drills with different attachments – a diamond dust drill with a pointed finish to clean the cuticle, a sharper tool to take off the dead skin around the edge of the nails, and a sandy textured tool to smooth. It sounds incredibly painful, but he's not drilling with those drills, he's just passing the attachments over the nails to smooth down the surface.

Bastien has a social conscience. He hasn't always just done the well-heeled feet of the jet-set. (His pedicures cost from £80, and even though they last for up to five weeks, we're not talking bargain basement here.) Once a week he would work with the homeless in Paris, whose feet were severely neglected. They're more neglected now, as he's stopped doing them, due to his clients' needs taking precedence, but it is an experience from which he learned a lot. 'One day I saw an ingrowing nail that went over the nail and back up underneath until it touched the toe. The man was homeless, and he'd never cut his nails.'

But despite his passion for feet, he is not averse to a little foot abuse. 'I love women in high heels,' he says. 'More than five centimetres for the foot is terrible because you put all the weight at the front of the foot. But high heels give a lovely shape to a woman's leg. And they're very good for business.'

Pedicure or podiatry?

Bastien explains: 'A pedicure deals with all the problems with the skin on the feet, like ingrowing nails, corns and callouses. Podiatry is about inverting things inside the shoes to correct the position. It's more about the architecture of the foot.'

Bastien's natural pedicure at home

The best time to do this is after a long bath, when the hard skin on the ball and heel of the foot is more likely to lift up. Using a pumice stone or file on wet feet, rub very gently over areas of hard skin in a circular motion. Dry the feet, then follow with a massage with an oil or foot cream to soothe any inflammation you may have created by rubbing and to improve circulation. If you massage your feet every night they will look great. ('If you say every night, that means you'll do it once a week.') Especially with younger people, massage is very effective – after a certain age your skin loses its elasticity. If you focus on the massage you will restore the fatty cushions of your feet, which are vital for the foot's overall shape and balance. Regular massage also means you can wear whatever shoes you want – more or less. Cut your nails straight across the toe in a square shape, then file. Never, repeat, never, cut down the side of the nail. It's asking for trouble. And never cut too short, otherwise the skin grows against the nail and creates an inflammation. Buff the nails with a chamois leather to help boost the circulation and give them a good shine.

What are the best shoes for your feet?

Not necessarily the ones you think. With some natural-looking shoes the arch is completely unnatural and not good for the foot. Put your hand inside the shoe and if you can't feel any seams or sudden arches it will be gentle enough for your foot. The front should be supple to accept the volume of the ground, and the back should be harder to support the ankle.

What is the best way to remove a corn?

Leave it to the professionals. You can do a lot of damage if you start fiddling about with it. The corn is an area of hard skin, normally on the toes, where the shoes have rubbed against them and created pressure. A point, like a nucleus, forms inside it. A professional will clean it, remove the hard skin with a scalpel, then remove the centre with a steel blade with a point. If you then do nothing, in about three weeks the corn will reappear. 'It's a great way for chiropodists or pedicurists to make money – imagine, if they get ten people a day with corns, voilà!' says Bastien. 'They'll be back three weeks later!' If, on the other hand, you do as Bastien does, which is to massage the skin with a foot cream by lifting up the skin of the corn and rolling it, you will prevent the skin from sticking to the bone and help restore the elasticity. 'Skin is the first defence against shoes – you are restoring the circulation of the blood.' Whatever you do, avoid chemical products on the feet. 'One of my clients burnt right through her skin – it took over a month to restore.'

Too hot, too cold

When your ankles are looking a little swollen either as the result of hot weather, pregnancy, or general fluid retention, drink lots of water and herbal teas, and bathe the feet and ankles in warm water with Epsom salts. If you suffer from feet like blocks of ice and you don't have a willing husband, boyfriend, girlfriend or small child to warm them up on, soak your feet in warm water with a pinch of mustard added for ten minutes.

What should you do about ingrowing toenails and corns?

Try to prevent them – the ultimate horror has to be having to go to hospital to have the whole nail removed. Toenails are very curved. When they grow, the nail grows round and rubs against the skin. The skin reacts and creates a corn. As soon as the nails grow, the corn will come back. See a professional to have the hard skin removed. Bastien then massages with oil and puts a small piece of cotton between the nail and the skin. 'What you're aiming for is to create a little distance between the nail and the skin. But you have to apply oil regularly and massage, otherwise the skin hardens again and catches the nail.'

What can you do to ease the pain of switching from winter shoes (worn with tights or socks) to summer sandals (barefoot)?

'You spend all winter in socks, and they keep your feet soft and protected,' says Bastien. 'Your skin just isn't prepared; it is thin because it has been cocooned. The only thing to do is to massage with oil regularly – not only will it prevent your skin from becoming dry and unsupple, but it will keep your circulation going when the first heat causes your feet to swell.' Something else that may be worth trying: rub a little cornflour on to your blister. It's said to help it heal.

What annoys Bastien

1 Cutting down the side of toenails. (Unless you want ingrowing nails.)
2 Leaving nail polish on for too long. The final word on lacquer is: 'It's like plastic. The nails dry out and grow in a different shape. A gap forms and the fungus grows.'

'Gardenia perfume ling'ring on a pillow . . .'
Bryan Ferry, 'These Foolish Things'

Chapter Six

HONEYSUCKLE AND CHAMPAGNE

I had borrowed a dress from the fashion department. It was a gorgeous slip of a thing, with a clever lining that held everything in, and a lace effect that sat comfortably over it. You had to be very careful taking it on and off in case the tiny sequins fell off – in fact, those were my fashion editor's parting words.

I had a bath, put on some make-up, went down to the lobby of the hotel, and joined the other thirty or so beauty journalists ready for the perfume launch. We were in Paris for the launch of Miracle by Lancôme, and the presentation of their new 'face', the actress Uma Thurman. There was a dinner, a fun one, followed by the launch itself, which for some reason involved acrobats shimmying up and down a pole. To my horror, one of the models – another 'face' for Lancôme, was wearing the same dress as me, only rather better.

The following day we were whisked off to the home of arch-perfumer Jean Paul Guerlain for the launch of Guerlain's new fragrance, Mahora. Here we were led from one small tent, into another enormous one, complete with its own sand dune, and special desert effects, all designed to help us get to grips with the concept of the new fragrance. One beauty editor was so overwhelmed she had an attack of the giggles. Afterwards there was a huge lunch, and then home we all came on Eurostar.

Perfume launches are legendary. They cost thousands and thousands of pounds. Some are still talked about ten years later – like the one in a converted air hangar, which had semi-naked girls floating on lily pads, with divers underneath propelling them along. For the public relations people launching them, they must be a nightmare. Just the logistics of having to get the right number of the right people to attend them is bad enough. Then there is the pressure of selling the fragrance itself. Most fragrances are launched just before Christmas in time to catch the Christmas market. This gives a fragrance a window of twelve weeks or so in which to sell. The shelf life of the average perfume is somewhere between three and five years. No wonder marketing teams go to such lengths to create the right concept, and then spend just as long working on the bottle design and the launch party.

There are now so many launches a year (it is not uncommon for a big fragrance house like Givaudan to launch over 1000 in one year, including some 'prestige' fragrances for design houses such as Yves Saint-Laurent) that, if I'm to be completely honest, it is hard to remember them all. Once, stuck in the airport at São Paulo with nothing to do except browse the duty free shop, I was astounded to see that in a relatively small space, crammed between alarm clocks and cigarettes, there was a huge display of hundreds of perfumes – many that I had never even heard of. With some, like Gabriela Sabatini's range, this wasn't surprising. A huge star in South America, her perfume range hadn't even launched in Europe. But others were from mainstream prestige fragrance houses; they were spin-offs of older fragrances, as well as completely new perfumes. I should be able to remember these.

There are two reasons why, over the last few years, perfume production seems to have increased so dramatically. First, we wear fragrance differently. Gone are the days when a woman would stay loyal to one perfume her whole life. We wear fragrances now that suit our mood, our wardrobe, the place we're going to. Second, spare a thought for those girls in department stores who have to sell perfumes. It can't be easy articulating the sense of smell, which is purely subjective. And if you only have a line of three different ones, it's even harder. The perfume companies know that in order to keep at the top, they need to keep having something new to sell. Which puts even more pressure on the perfumers to come up with the right combinations.

Pierre Bourdon is a perfumer with a wife who, like me, is called Kathleen. I say this, because ever since we met years ago at the launch of a fragrance he had created for the natural beauty company L'Occitane, it has been a common connection. It has meant that every time I call him for interviews he has made time for me. His wife, whom I have never met, is English, and Bourdon, a Frenchman, also speaks perfect English, which is another reason for the connection – my husband is French too. Bourdon is at the front-line of fragrance. You won't have heard of him – he's the guy in the lab, mixing and blending until he comes up with the right concoction for someone else to then stick their name on. In my view he is something of a genius, because he has collaborated on one of the most beautiful perfumes in the world: Feminité du Bois by Shiseido, which was created by Serge Lutens in 1992. Like most true perfumers I speak to, Bourdon is passionate about perfume. 'Fragrance is about love, passion, sex and everything that is very exciting in life!' And yet, this time when I called him, perhaps he was just having a bad day, but he sounded almost disenchanted with the business of perfumery. 'I'm very worried about the future of this industry,' he said 'We are experiencing a crisis that I have never experienced in my thirty-one years of working in it. It's very, very bad. And everyone knows that it's because of a lack of innovation. I just wish the big groups would take risks again because everything smells the same. If they don't, they will melt like ice in the sun – they are already experiencing drops of 40–50 per cent in the States.'

As an example of a perfume that is truly innovative, he singles out Angel, by Thierry Mugler – a blend of bergamot and jasmine as the top notes, dewberry and honey as the middle, and patchouli, vanilla and chocolate as the soul. Now I personally hate Angel. I cannot abide it. I think it is strong, overpowering and sickly sweet, and I feel irritated and tense whenever I am around someone wearing it. If someone came to me for a job interview who was perfect in every way, I would probably not employ them if they wore this fragrance, or I would have to ask them to give it up. But I still appreciate Angel as a fragrance. I can see why others like it. It is distinctive, it isn't bland. And at least it provokes a reaction, at least it makes me feel *something*.

'Angel is a difficult fragrance,' says Bourdon. 'No one would have wanted it except Thierry Mugler. It was small when it started, but little by little the most difficult fragrance became a bestseller, even in France, which is a conservative country. Not only does it mean something the first time it is sold, but it is so innovative, so different, it has true character. Knowing the success of Angel, every head of marketing should say, 'Okay, now I know that to be successful I need to be provocative and take a risk.' But no, they just want copies of things.'

This explains why shortly after Angel launched, we suddenly had a spate of vanilla-based fragrances. I remember there was a time not so long ago when every fragrance launched claimed to smell of the ocean, following the launch of the hugely successful CKOne by Calvin Klein. There are even machines, commonly used by some fragrance houses, that can break down the exact components of a fragrance and recreate it in its entirety – not that they'd want to make one exactly the same, because who would want it? But you can see how, with the right twists and turns, suddenly you have Ocean Breeze, Ocean Wave, Ocean Whatever (with apologies if there are fragrances with names like this already in existence). This must be how trends start.

'No one decides on trends – it's a collective type of work,' says Bourdon. 'You invent something good and you start a trend, and this is a positive aspect, but when it gets copied by everyone . . . by the time the trend finishes it's very sad. Everything smells the same and the customers don't like it. When Opium came out everything smelt like Opium; when Giorgio came out, everything was about tuberose. There are less and less products that tell a story – they are all a bit like American movies. Once you've seen one, you've seen them all. They are marketing products with each scene tested to check it will suit all the consumers and will sell.'

If all of this makes Bourdon sound like a huge cynic, he's not. He became a perfumer after studying economics and politics left him a little cold. 'I realised I was more interested in art than anything else, and I thought perfume was a happy medium, linked with business, but also with an art, the art of perfumery. My father worked at Christian Dior and I had been exposed to perfume as a child, so very early on I smelled blotters and things like that, but I never thought I would become a perfumer. My father was delighted.'

He came to work on Feminité du Bois almost by chance. Serge Lutens approached Quest, the company he was working for at the time, and invited four perfumers to Marrakesh. Bourdon was not one of them. The creative genius behind the make-up range for Shiseido, and a huge perfume aficionado, Serge had an idea: 'I want a fragrance that smells like a woodshop in Marrakesh.' The four perfumers came up with a rough base of woody notes, using cedarwood, but then it was up to Bourdon, back in Paris, to work with Serge on converting this roughness into something sophisticated.

'He is a true creator,' Bourdon says, 'and I was really the illustrator of what he is, putting into practice his ideas. It took about three to four months of him coming to the lab at least once a week, and we'd smell what was done, work a little bit more, and it's what I would call a 'small step policy', trying to convince him that it wasn't too far away from what he wanted but more sophisticated than the original. It was completely his own idea, but I put my soul and feelings into it. I have good memories: he is a true gentleman, with great respect for the work that was done.'

Soul. Feelings. How can you put 'soul and feelings' into a perfume? 'Most of the time it's unconscious,' says Bourdon. 'But others will recognise a style which is mine. What do you call a style? It's what Marcel Proust would call "La Patrie Interieur" – the Inside Country, the fatherland . . . In Feminité du Bois there is my own music. Most of the symphony is the music of Serge Lutens, but I did the arrangement. All the spices, which are typical of Feminité du Bois – cinnamon, cardamom, clove – they're all Arabic. And they all come from an old product of perfumer Edmond Roudnitska's, which is L'Eau d'Hermès.'

Bourdon knows when he's created a winner. 'If you wear it yourself and you get a comment, you can be sure you've created a bestseller. And when you wear it and you have no comments, you can be sure you have to work on it again.'

Our conversation is over. Bourdon has to go. And then he says something a little sad: 'I've been fighting now for so long for real creativity, and almost no one listens to me.' But a perfumer's passion never dies: 'I'm working on many exciting things, so hopefully I will be ready when the industry decides to be . . . a little more innovative.'

PIERRE BOURDON'S TOP INNOVATIVE FRAGRANCES

If Pierre Bourdon were giving out awards for fragrance innovation, all of these would be winning prizes. If you want something truly original, go try them:

Alliage 'This is what I would call a fragrance for perfumers: it is a great fragrance and very innovative,' says Bourdon of this 1972 green, spicy perfume, created by Estée Lauder.

Angel Created by Olivier Cresp and Yves de Chiris of Quest International in 1992, this sexy scent was inspired by the designer Thierry Mugler's love of stars. The perfume started with the star concept and the fabulous blue-glass bottle, and broke the mould at the time by mixing fruits and flowers with the more unusual notes of patchouli, vanilla, coumarin, chocolate and caramel.

Cool Water Man 'This was a fragrance which no one wanted and was sleeping in a drawer,' says Bourdon, who created it for Davidoff. Made in 1988, it was a first in 'new freshness' as far as olfactory families go. The top notes are zesty bergamot, peppermint, aromatic lavender and rosemary, green galbanum and pineapple. The heart is violet, jasmine, honeysuckle and orange blossom. Woody notes of sandalwood, cedar and oakmoss, along with coriander and juniper, form the base.

Diorissimo 'This is so simple, and yet it is magnificent.' The lily of the valley was the lucky charm of Christian Dior, and happened to be growing in the garden of arch-perfumer Edmond Roudnitska. His genius interpretation is what makes this mono-perfume, launched in 1956, succeed where others have failed:

it's the combination of lily of the valley buds, with a middle note of lily of the valley and boronia and amaryllis, as well as jasmine and sandalwood.

Fahrenheit Created by Jean-Louis Sieuzac for Christian Dior in 1988, this men's floral-woody fragrance uses notes from hawthorn and honeysuckle, with a base of sandalwood and cedar.

Giorgio The fragrance of the original fashion store in Beverly Hills, California, the packaging matched the yellow and white awnings, and was a huge hit in the 1980s. Its key notes are jasmine, gardenia and orange flower, combined with sandalwood, patchouli and camomile.

Mitsouko 'It's full of mystery, and is a favourite for sentimental reasons. It smells like women would have smelt before the First World War.' Created by Jacques Guerlain in 1919, it has fresh, fruity top notes of bergamot, with lemon, mandarin, neroli and peach, a floral middle of jasmine, rose and ylang-ylang, a touch of spice with cloves, and an oak moss and musk base.

Obsession for Women 'A great thing.' This Calvin Klein fragrance was a huge hit when it launched in 1985, and was all about passion. The top notes are mandarin, bergamot, the middle notes jasmine, orange blossom, sandalwood, vetiver and spices, and the base, amber, oakmoss, incense and musk.

Opium 'This was a statement, although for me it's a bit close to Youth Dew [Estée Lauder]. Yves Saint-Laurent's marketing for this fragrance caused an outrage in the 1970s when billboards went up featuring a naked young Yves. The current ads, with a naked Sophie Dahl, have been no less controversial. The fragrance is an Oriental type, with mandarins, cloves, coriander, lily of the valley, rose and jasmine, and a base of cedarwood and sandalwood. It was created by Jean-Louis Sieuzac and Jean Amic.

Samsara 'A great fragrance and very elegant – a true statement.' Jean Paul Guerlain brought out this amber fragrance in 1989. Sandalwood and jasmine are its top notes, with a middle layer of rose, narcissus, violet and orris, and a base with amber, vanilla and tonka.

Youth Dew 'This was certainly something outstanding.' Estée Lauder's Oriental perfume was first sold in 1952, but it's still a bestseller. It's a blend of orange, spices, rose, ylang-ylang and jasmine, with a base of amber.

Edmond who?

If you want to look like you know about perfume in just a few minutes, it's vital to drop the name Edmond Roudnitska into your conversation. Born in 1905, he is the perfumer's perfumer, having created Diorissimo, Diorella and Eau Sauvage for Christian Dior, as well as Femme for Rochas, and L'Eau d'Hermès for Hermès. He was one of Pierre Bourdon's teachers. He died in 1997.

Feminité du Bois by Shiseido, launched in 1992, was created by Serge Lutens, with the help of Pierre Bourdon. The dominant note is Absolute of Atlas cedar, which is a yellowish oil with a rich, warm and woody fragrance. It is backed up by Moroccan orange blossom and Turkish rose, with peach, honey essence, beeswax and violet as middle notes, and a base of cardamom, cinnamon, clove, musk and vanilla. It's the kind of fragrance only a woman who is sure of herself will wear.

GREAT FRAGRANCE STORIES NO 1: MITSOUKO BY GUERLAIN

Key notes: oak moss, ambergris, vetiver, peach, spices, lilac and bergamot

The story behind one of Pierre Bourdon's favourite fragrances, Mitsouko, was inspired by the heroine in Claude Farrère's 1919 novel La Bataille. *It came shortly after*

Puccini's Madame Butterfly, *at a time when Europe was fascinated by all things Eastern. The chiefs of Russia and Japan were at war over who would control Manchuria. In desperation, the Russian Tsar dispatched the entire Baltic fleet to his Vladivostok naval base in readiness for a final attack. In command of the Japanese fleet was Admiral Togo, who was accompanied by his young, devastatingly beautiful wife, Mitsouko. A British officer fell passionately in love with her, and they embarked on a dangerous affair, while meanwhile war raged on all around them.*

The Admiral knew of the affair all along, but knew he had to focus on the war ahead. He ordered the Japanese fleet to engage with the Baltic fleet, and thirty-six hours later, all but twelve of the Russian warships were sunk, captured or run aground. The Japanese had completely crushed them. Jacques Guerlain created this fragrance in honour of the young girl.

Opposite the Cock and Bottle pub, just around the corner from the Church of St Mary of the Angels, and near the fancy boutiques of Westbourne Grove, London W11, is a small shop called Miller Harris. It sells perfumes. Not very many of them – they produce only thirteen fragrances and essences – but enough to have a loyal following and a thriving bespoke section, to say nothing of consultancies left, right and centre for perfume companies whose names we shall never know because they want you to think they made them all by themselves. It is the brainchild of Lyn Harris, a young perfumer who set up her own shop after working from a small laboratory at home for years. When I say *young* perfumer, she's probably about my age, but somehow in perfumery that still seems young. I imagine perfumers to bring years of experience, to have a thousand stories of travel, women, wine and song to bring to their fragrances, and it's hard when someone as gamine as Lyn comes along to shake off that image.

Which doesn't mean to say she's any less passionate about perfume. 'On my visits to Grasse to buy my essences, it's really refreshing that I am perceived as a younger perfumer even though I'm surrounded by an older generation,' she says. 'But I know I wouldn't be where I am today without them. Their knowledge is phenomenal. The guy who helps me there is about ready to retire, but he is inspired by my passion and by what I want to do. If I can take the industry forward and keep the light burning . . . well, that would be something.'

She shows me around her laboratory, which is in the basement of the shop. She is slight but not frail, pretty, with clothes that are casually chic and a slight tan. She looks like the kind of girl who comes alive in sunshine. Her eyes are clear and bright. I am surprised that the laboratory is so small, and then I remember this is not someone who is churning out thousands of perfumes every year. Even so, there are hundreds of small brown bottles with black lids and white labels, as well as phial upon phial of chemically produced smells which smell surprisingly nice. There is a computer, from which she orders supplies – raw essences and aroma chemicals, a cluttered desk, and a view on to a small garden at the back. 'You know, there are thousands and thousands of aroma chemicals,' she says, giving me some to try. 'All you can do is filter through them. I have 500 raw materials alone in my lab, the ones that are my favourites.'

Harris tells me how the raw materials get from the fields in France to her laboratory. 'It's really quite wonderful . . . A farmer comes with his crop in the morning. He leaves his goods, which depend on what's in season. The director of the factory tests it. He has a good look at it, and then they start the process of extracting the essence from the petals. Let's say this is Jasmine Absolute . . . You know, I have seen the jasmine fields in Grasse in summer, and they're amazing . . .

'The process of extraction is called *enfleurage*. They take trays of vegetable fat – it used to be animal fat – they lay the petals on top, tray upon tray upon tray. Then they leave it for months so that the fat absorbs the jasmine juices, and then it is distilled.' She pauses, looking at me to check I have understood, and then says, 'I tell you what, let's see if this book explains it any better.' A huge volume – a perfume guidebook, obviously meant as a text book for students – is thrust in front of me, and Lyn marks out the passage that is relevant.

'In order to isolate and concentrate this matter, the flowers are extracted with a hydrocarbon solution, usually petroleum ether. The petroleum ether extract is evaporated and the evaporation residue is extracted with alcohol. In turn, the alcohol is moved from this extract, and what is left is called Jasmin Absolute from chassis. This is actually a by-product to the *enfleurage* process and the annual amount of available chassis-absolute is obviously very small. Furthermore it is constantly decreasing with the lessening use of the *enfleurage* method.'

I decide I prefer Harris's explanation. She continues: 'The minute you use a lot of heat you destroy the molecular structures, so when you're distilling it has to be a gentle process, heating up the fat very gently and then passing the alcohol over it. The juice is then sent to the perfumer.

'But anything that comes from Grasse now is highly expensive. Only the niche brands like L'Artisan Parfumeur, Annick Goutal, ourselves and a few others can afford such essences. Chanel is one of the few remaining mainstream companies to have its own field there. Once I went to see some tuberose fields. There is a farmer who has two fields of them, and his whole life is devoted to producing and growing the tuberose. I would go morning and night to watch it being picked because it's at these times of the day that the scent is heightened. It's very sexist – only the women can pick the flowers because they have gentler hands!'

It's not just the ingredients from Grasse that are expensive. Olivier Creed, who makes made-to-measure fragrances for a very select clientele, and whose family house (founded in 1760) has in the past created perfumes for Princess Grace of Monaco, Marlene Dietrich, Natalie Wood and Ava Gardner, once told me that he spends £4–5000 for a kilo of Tibetan musk and £7000 for a kilo of iris. Rose Bulgarie is incredibly expensive – he once made a fragrance that was 70 per cent of this essence alone. He charges around £4000 for a bespoke fragrance; Lyn Harris charges significantly less – around £1200 – but once you know that most of the ingredients they use are of the highest quality, you can see why it's not £29.99 with a free washbag thrown in for good measure.

Synthetic notes might be cheaper, and indeed some mass-produced fragrances contain nothing but synthetic notes, but sometimes they are also essential. 'Can a synthetic jasmine be as good as a pure jasmine? I don't think so,' says Pierre Bourdon. 'A minute touch of a pure jasmine has something a synthetic cannot bring. But some synthetics are better than naturals, like woody notes. Muguet (lily of the valley) and mimosa are much better as synthetics. In the case of muguet, we have never been able to produce a natural one.'

Aroma chemicals provide an important fantasy element to perfumery. 'A scientific perfumer will analyse the structures and play around with the 300 or so constituents of jasmine, creating something like Headione, which is a highly used chemical,' explains Lyn Harris. 'Your naturals, which are today used less and less in commercial perfumery because of the price, are needed because they bring integrity and soul to your fragrances. But aroma chemicals bring life, fantasy and creativity.'

Her bespoke clients, of course, aren't expected to pick their way through this infinite muddle of synthetics and naturals. 'I can tell just by being with a client, learning about their personality and getting a picture in my head, what they really want.' They'll sit downstairs with her in the laboratory, and, depending on how developed their nose is, will either bring ideas to her, or rely on her totally to interpret their passions and desires, their anxieties and weaknesses. 'I'm a good listener,' she says. 'Sometimes I talk, sometimes people talk at me. I do love people, I want to understand them. Every client I have to some extent helps me evolve as a more creative person. Some are very demanding, others are totally respectful of what you do. But you know, usually the first trial that you do is the one people go for. And if you play around too much you lose something.'

Back upstairs in the shop I see how intuitive she really is. She picks up a beautiful bottle and hands it to me. Her bottles are clear glass, with an intricate swirling floral design picked out in black. 'Here, try this,' she says. 'You'll like it.' I take a big sniff, and for a moment am right outside the house where I grew up in Kent. It was Victorian, with a black trellis over the front door, which in summer was intertwined with sweet-smelling honeysuckle. There were big bumble bees buzzing around, the kind you don't see any more. It was a favourite spot for my father to take pictures of us, so all our photos taken here have us in party dresses or with big bows in our hair. How fantastic it must be to be able to transport someone to a happy place just like that!

This fragrance smells like honeysuckle with champagne. How does she know I will like it? She shoots me a big smile. 'I just do.'

GREAT FRAGRANCE STORIES NO 2: SHALIMAR BY GUERLAIN

Key notes: bergamot, rose, jasmine, vanilla, iris, tonka bean

Jacques and Raymond Guerlain were first told this story of Mumtaz Mahal and the Mogul emperor by a maharajah they met in Paris. As a tribute, they created the fragrance Shalimar.

More than 300 years ago, Shah Jahan was the third Mogul Emperor of India. As was the tradition, he had many wives, but there was only one whom he really loved. Her name was Mumtaz Mahal. The Shah was extraordinarily rich, and had conquered empires the length and breadth of the world, but he lived for her and her alone. They would spend many happy hours in the gardens of Shalimar set around the palace in which they lived. The gardens were full of pools with crystal fountains, marble terraces, and fragrant blossoms and rare birds were brought from the four corners of the world. But then Mumtaz died while giving birth to their fourteenth child. Shah Jahan was so distraught that his hair turned white overnight. He would burst into tears at the mention of her name. He resolved to build a palace in her memory and set thousands of men to work. Fourteen years later, the palace was completed, and he named it the Taj Mahal.

LYN HARRIS'S TOP INNOVATIVE FRAGRANCES

Chanel No 5 Created by Coco Chanel (the first couturier to produce a perfume) with her then lover, the perfumer Ernest Beaux. This was the first perfume to use aldehydes, which give a zing to the ylang-ylang and neroli, the floral heart of jasmine and rose, and the woody base notes of sandalwood and vetiver. The bottle is just as iconic as the fragrance – it was designed by Sem, a French artist, and was chosen to reflect the simplicity of Chanel's clothes.

Diorissimo by Christian Dior – see p.147.

Eau de Ciel by Annick Goutal was created in 1985. Inspired by 'a walk in a cut wheatfield in the south of France', it's the perfect summery perfume, with tender notes of rosewood from Brazil, and violet and iris from Florence.

Eau Sauvage This men's eau de toilette started a huge trend for citrus fragrances in 1966, and was created by Edmond Roudnitska for Christian Dior. Bergamot, lemon and basil, backed up by jasmine and patchouli, with a base of oak moss, was a magic formula that took everyone's favourite eau de cologne to a higher level.

Femme Created by Edmond Roudnitska for Rochas, this was launched in 1944 as a tribute to Marcel Rochas's wife. It's a classic chypre perfume with fruity top notes of peach, plum and apricot, a floral middle note of jasmine and rose underlined by patchouli and amber, and a base of oak moss and vanilla. Rochas collaborated with Lalique to create the bottle.

Gardenia Passion by Annick Goutal was created in 1989 and is a mix of tuberose, with gardenia and orange blossom, and a base of underlying moss and jasmine.

Mitsouko by Jacques Guerlain – see p.148.

That honeysuckle fragrance. What was it?

One of Lyn Harris's special concoctions that is available only from the shop itself, Fleurs de Matin by Miller Harris, was inspired by the dew that falls on morning flowers. Smelling of honeysuckle, with jasmine, neroli, galbanum and basil leaves, it has a special sparkle thanks to the addition of grapefruit and lemon leaves. It is completely gorgeous.

GREAT FRAGRANCE STORIES NO. 3: JOY BY JEAN PATOU

Key notes: Bulgarian rose, tuberose, ylang-ylang, jasmine, may rose

Jean Patou was a flamboyant couturier who lived in Paris in the early 1900s. Fond of music and parties, he worked as hard as he played. He was handsome, and set about changing the clothing customs of his companions, making sportswear, bathing suits and other things for them to enjoy. He was a bit of a ladies' man.

But behind all this, he was also a little sad, having spent four years fighting in the trenches of the First World War as an infantryman. This nightmare had left him more determined to make the most of his life.

When the world's banks and financial institutions crashed, he and his friends had to fight for their survival and saw their lifestyles seriously cramped. Patou decided to cheer them all up, and set upon the idea of giving them something so precious they would be filled with joy. He journeyed to Grasse and took with him his favourite lady friend, Elsa Maxwell. They arrived at the house of a perfumer (Henri Almeras) – renowned for his talent and excitable temperament – who presented them with a fragrance to smell. They were entranced, but were told that its cost was so exorbitant that it would be impossible to reproduce. For Patou this was like a red rag to a bull. Determined to have it, he ordered enough bottles of the precious essence to send to all his friends who could no longer afford to travel to see him. He called it 'Joy; the costliest perfume in the world'.

What made Lyn Harris want to be a perfumer?

'Even as a child, my olfactory memory was developed. I used to drive my mother mad. I wouldn't go to certain people's houses because I didn't like the smell. I started my career working with essential oils because I loved the psychological benefits and the way they worked. I went to perfume school in Paris to learn about the chemical side. I studied with a woman I'd previously only read about: Monique Schlienger, who was the creator for Annick Goutal. I worked in my local town's fragrance shop. I've always known I had the ability to create – perfume was always a part of my life.'

We don't always have a Lyn Harris to hand to help us choose a fragrance that fits. But if you write about beauty, you do nearly always have Roja Dove to hand, and his is a hand that is well worth shaking. Roja is a true dandy of the twenty-first century – a larger-than-life *bon viveur*, with a mischievous glimmer in his eye and a passion that goes beyond all others for perfume. Roja brings perfume alive. They didn't know what to call him when he worked at Guerlain, so he gave himself a title, 'professeur des parfums', which was appropriate as he wheeled in beauty editor after beauty editor to teach them about the subject, and now, even as an independent consultant, this is what he is still known as. It's a dull day in the office, until he pitches up in a crushed purple velvet jacket carrying a Louis Vuitton bag to show me his latest line: bespoke fragrances. We chat about the product a bit, and then one thing leads to another, and the question I have been puzzling over for a while finds the best person to answer it. 'How do you choose a fragrance?'

I should know this. And yet the more fragrances I smell, the more bottles I look at, the more laminated folders I read of completely nonsensical gibberish about notes and feelings and memories and places and God knows what – just *anything* to make me write about the damn thing – leave me feeling confused and empty. I love lots of them! But I still can't find the right one for me.

'How do you choose a fragrance, Roja?' And he warms straight away to the subject, as ever. 'First of all, you have to understand why we respond to fragrances the way we do. When we're born, the part of the brain that deals with odour is empty, and the first ten or twenty years of life tell you what you like and what you don't like.' I've seen this with my babies. How is it that changing a nappy is utter hell for me and my husband, but there they lie, giggling and gurgling, rolling this way and that, grumbling and whingeing when they get bored, and kicking their little toes dangerously near the offending article? 'Bad' smells just don't bother them.

'Smell is the most primitive of all the senses – people say you can smell death, or fear! Yet, we forget this in an industry that churns so many fragrances out – and I'm not knocking it for that, I think it's great – but we do take our sense of smell for granted. We talk about beautiful works of art, a marvellous chef, a classic wine, but it's very rare that we will eulogise over this sense . . .' He senses I am anxious to get on with the subject in hand. 'Anyway, how to choose a fragrance . . . Well, unless something really significant happens in your life, like a divorce or a death, your basic odour profile, what you build upon from birth, will stay with you until you die. It's as unique as a fingerprint. All you have to do is discover the basic blocks of odour that you relate to positively.'

This doesn't sound simple at all to me. What on earth is a 'block of odour'? A bar of soap?

'I've developed a methodology over the years to discover these basic blocks of odour,' Dove says. 'At its simplest level, perfume falls into one of three categories: floral, chypre and oriental. Then, once you've found which family you favour, you go into the sub-categories, and from the sub-categories you go into the tiny nuances. It's all done through memory association. And when I'm trying to find the right fragrance for someone, I don't tell them what it is until afterwards.'

The reason he won't say boils down to the fact that we are all complete and utter perfume snobs, and easily influenced by bottles, marketing campaigns – indeed, everything except the smell itself. There are other more practical pointers. For example, something so obvious and yet we all do it . . .

'Never wear a fragrance when you go to buy one,' says Dove. 'The number of people who come already wearing one . . . And never go with a friend. They have their own olfactory fingerprint, and what is good for them is not good for you. It takes a very strong character to say, "I don't care what you think, I think it's lovely."'

'Always smell perfumes on smelling strips, never on the skin itself,' he continues. 'It is a huge misconception that it will smell differently on skin. Skin will only modify a fragrance slightly, it will bring a fragrance to life. I hear time after time, "My skin's acidic," and I always say, "Well, good for you." Your skin is meant to have an acid mantle, otherwise you'd die from bacteria.

'Give yourself time. Really, you should allow yourself a day. You need time to compare perfume families to find out which one you really like. Once you've found one you like, spray yourself with it, not just on your wrists but all over, then walk away and live with it for the day. You know, a perfume is just like a lover, you only know whether it will work when you've spent the night with them.'

And sometimes, I think to myself, not even then.

PERFUME-OLOGY: WHAT DOES IT ALL MEAN?

Nigel Groom, who is a friend of my mother's, has written an extraordinarily detailed book on perfumes (*The Perfume Handbook*, published by Chapman & Hall) listing all the different ingredients in perfumes, and even including some ancient recipes. Here is a shortened explanation of the three different families Roja was talking about:

Chypre The Ancient Romans made a perfume in Cyprus (Chypre in French) that was based on storax (the inner bark of a small tree, sometimes used in incense), labdanum (a sweet resin) and calamus (a sweet-smelling reed), which gave it a distinctively heady and Oriental aroma. It continued to be manufactured in Italy well into the Middle Ages, and was produced in France with oak moss as a base. The main ingredients of a chypre perfume now are oak moss, patchouli, labdanum or clary sage, with the addition of flowery notes such as rose jasmine, and a sweet note such as bergamot or lemon.

Floral A perfume with a predominantly floral note. Probably half of all perfumes sold today fall into this category.

Oriental This is the type of perfume that, as you would expect, is reminiscent of the spices and balms reflecting the exotic character of the East. Commonly found ingredients include vanilla, cumin, amber and sandalwood, musk, civet, castor, cloves, cinnamon and nutmeg.

GREAT FRAGRANCE STORIES NO. 4: FEMME BY ROCHAS

Key notes: bergamot, spice, peach, prune, Bulgarian rose immortelle, jasmine, ylang-ylang, ambergris, musk, oak moss and sandalwood

Hélène had hair that shone like spiderwebs, and was the favourite model of Marcel Rochas, the1940s' couturier. She lived in Paris and met him when she was eighteen. Immensely sophisticated, Rochas travelled the world making costly gowns for the world's most beautiful women. He was infatuated with the female form, making clothes with shapely shoulders, nipped-in waists, curved hips, and lingerie from the finest Chantilly lace. But when he saw Hélène he was entranced. Her tiny waist and rounded hips seemed to him to be the ultimate in femininity, and he decided she was the perfect woman to model the latest collection of hats he had created. He fell in love with her, and asked her to marry him. She became his wife, companion, muse and mother of his two children.

On the day of their wedding, Hélène found among the gifts a present from him. Nestling in lace lingerie was a curved crystal flacon containing a perfume made just for her by Edmond Roudnitska. Marcel said, 'I wanted to create a perfume just for you.' He called the perfume Femme. It was launched publicly in 1944.

What's so special about perfume? Roja Dove's first fragrance memory

'When I was very young, about six or seven years old, my mother came to kiss me goodnight. She was on her way to a cocktail party and had on a gold lamé dress. The light was on behind her on the landing. I could smell her face powder, her perfume, she was metamorphosed into a goddess. I told a perfumer about this once, and I happened to mention the name of the perfume she used to wear. Years later, I was sitting in a hotel in New York, and I put a bit of perfume on my hand and smelt it, and the moment I smelt it I knew it was my mother, and the tears just kept pouring . . . Sometimes I think the industry has lost that a little. The fragrance was L'Aimant by Coty, but the original one – the formulas have now been altered.'

How should you store your fragrance?

I have given my mother loads of perfumes over the years, but nothing will replace her favourite, and the one my father used to give her: Fidji by Guy Laroche – a classic floral, created in 1966, with top notes of rose, ylang-ylang, jasmine, iris and tuberose, with spices, cloves and aldehydes underpinned by a base of sandalwood, patchouli and Peruvian balsam. But she's still proud of her new acquisitions. She thinks they make her look fantastically glamorous, so she displays them on a glass shelf in the bathroom. 'They'll get ruined by the sun!' I say. 'But, darling, they look so gorgeous!' she replies. In case she ever reads this, this is what she should be doing: keep your perfumes somewhere cool and dark, and lying flat, like a vintage wine. They'll keep a better seal that way, and if it's a good one, your fragrance will not only age well, but will improve over time.

ROJA DOVE'S TOP INNOVATIVE FRAGRANCES

Ambre Sultan 'It's very unusual – a non-mainstream perfume that is truly creative. It suggests a slight exoticism, and it helps us to dream a bit.' Created by Serge Lutens in 2000, it has amber, tree resins and patchouli, and was inspired by a piece of amber offered as a gift to Serge Lutens on his first trip to Marrakesh in 1968.

Bal à Versailles 'It has always been a slightly enigmatic perfume. It's available, and then it disappears. Its formula is fiendishly expensive, and however hard it is to get hold of, it has never lost its devotees. It is luscious and sensual, and makes me think of hugging someone wearing cashmere . . .' Created in 1962 by Jean Desprez, the notes are jasmine, vanilla, musk, civet and orris.

Calèche 'It's a very disciplined perfume, with the merest whisper of sensuality. Hermès took a risk with it: the top structure is completely magnificent, but it doesn't last. They hoped women would nonetheless find it so exquisite that they would be enticed back.' Created in 1992, the key notes are citrus and bergamot, orange and jasmine, with aldehydes to give it a cheerful fizz; rose and ylang-ylang for sensuality.

Le Dix 'It's as frothy and refined as a glass of champagne. It's as soft as a woman's skin.' Created in 1947 by Balenciaga, it's a classic aldehydic floral based on jasmine, ylang-ylang and rose, with a lot of woods in the base to give it warmth: sandalwood, vetiver, patchouli, vanilla and musk.

L'Eau d'Issey 'It was the first time the oceanic note entered perfumery. It was a new direction in fragrance.' Created in 1992 by Jacques Cavallier for Issey Miyake, with a modern, beautiful bottle by Fabien Baron, the watery floral has lotus, freesia, cyclamen and rose water; peony, carnation and tuberose, osmanthus, amber-seed and musk.

L'Heure Bleue 'It's a very romantic image. I imagine a French woman, slipping away in the distance, and this is the perfume that would linger in the air. It is hedonisitc and opulent, but not decadent.' Created in 1912 by Jacques Guerlain, the head is a fresh bergamot and aniseed, with a heart of carnation, orange blossom, heliotrope, Bulgarian rose and tuberose; and a base of iris, vanilla and musk.

Les Larmes Sacrées de Thèbes 'The extreme use of balsams in this perfume makes it very unusual. It nods back to the origin of perfumery when it was a rich and luxurious commodity that belonged only to kings and queens. The perfumer was given no commercial restraints.' Created by Baccarat in 1999, it has gum resins, frankincense, vanilla, a little orris, spice, jasmine and rose.

Miss Dior 'It's bright and breezy, with a fabulously rude and animalistic base. It's all about naughtiness underneath.' Created for Christian Dior by Jean Carles and Paul Vacher in 1947, its head is gardenia, galbanum, clary sage and aldehydes; the middle is jasmine, rose, neroli, iris and lily of the valley; and its base is patchouli, oak moss, sandalwood, vetiver and leather.

Mitsouko by Jacques Guerlain – see p. 148. 'Because I think it is the quintessential French perfume – it is sensual, while being very refined, and I love the strict discipline of the formula.'

Nuit de Noel 'It sums up for me the anticipation of festivities, the cool crispness of being outside when it's icy, and peering in through the window and seeing something warm, entrancing. I've worn it every Christmas Eve since I was an adult, and think it's quite magical that there is a perfume that exists for just one night of the year.' Created by Caron in 1922, the top notes are jasmine, ylang-ylang and May rose, the middle is violet leaves, lily of the valley, iris, Mousse de Saxe (a wild animalistic note, said to smell like 'the scent of a tiger's lair') and tuberose, and the base is sandalwood, vetiver and Mousse de Saxe again.

Tabac Blond 'This perfume broke all the rules, mainly because its creator, Ernest Daltroff, had never been formally trained as a perfumer. The idea was that it would induce a slightly narcotic state, taking as its inspiration the opium that was used in the cigarettes of the 1910s and 1920s. I love the warmth of the fragrance, and believe it to be one of the most underrated fragrances in the world.' Created by Caron in 1919, it has strong notes of tobacco and leather.

Vol de Nuit 'It was the first time the so-called green note was used in a perfume. It has the contrast between the dynamic freshness of its opening and the soft, powdery sensuality of its drydown. It's a perfume connoisseur's perfume.' Created in 1933 by Jacques and Pierre Guerlain, it was inspired by the story of the same name by the French aviator and poet Antoine de Saint-Exupéry. The key notes are vanilla, jonquil, spices, oak moss, galbanum, sandalwood and violet.

'Exercise is bunk. If you are healthy, you don't need it. If you are sick, you shouldn't take it.'
Henry Ford (1863–1947)

'If I said you had a beautiful body would you hold it against me?'
Dr Hook

'I must, I must, I must improve my bust.'
Anon.

Chapter Seven
THE CRAB WITH SPINNING EYES

I am in Cuba. The photographer is driving me from the airport to the hotel before we embark on a week's shooting for all the summer issues of *Tatler* magazine. 'What are the models like?' I ask, having seen only pictures of the girls, who have themselves arrived from Paris only a few hours before. 'Clarissa has long legs, she is beautiful, she is tanned, with boy's hips and absolutely no breasts. Daria has perfect breasts, just like a teenager's, but her bottom is not so good.'

I laugh to myself. If anyone could hear this conversation they would think he was a misogynist and that I was some Nazi anti-feminist. For the record, he is not, and neither am I. But sometimes attuned to the objective, graphic descriptions of women that I hear every time I do a shoot, I do wonder how we became so obsessed with the perfect body, particularly when the bodies in question are pretty perfect in the flesh. 'So I think,' he continues, 'we need both girls for the body story, and I can clean anything up afterwards on the computer.'

Cuba is no place for anyone with a few worries about body shape. The women we see in just a few days are all tall, long-legged, and they can do this thing with their bottoms when they dance that . . . well, suffice to say, it wouldn't be out of place in a lap-dancing club. If Cuba is a nightmare, add to that being on a trip with models when you've had not just one but two babies in the last three years, and you'll understand why I'm never very anxious to strip off and have a swim on one of the rare occasions when I'm near a beach and I have time between shots. I'm not the only one. Suddenly, our super-slim make-up artist really doesn't fancy a swim; my assistant really doesn't want to get her hair wet. The keen swimmers are the photographer (male) and the hairstylist (male).

When it comes down to it, looking good on the beach is a problem reserved exclusively for women. Men just don't care. This is a conversation I have with my husband on a regular basis, usually while dressing or undressing:

Him: (look of distaste) 'What are you going to do about your stomach?'
Me: 'What are you going to do about yours? At least I can blame mine on two babies. What's your excuse? Guinness?'
Him: 'Mine doesn't matter.'
Me: 'Why's that?'
Him: 'Because I'm a man.'
Me: 'So what?'
Him: 'Well, I don't care about mine. You're a woman, it's different.'
Me: 'Well, maybe I don't care either.'
Him: 'You have to care, you're a woman!'

How do you argue with that (without being abusive)? I do care about my stomach. And my bust. I also care about my bottom. And my thighs. But I'll be damned if it has anything whatsoever to do with what he thinks about them.

In Cuba, I watch what the models eat – not in a supervisory capacity, you understand, but purely to find out if they have any eating disorders, or something I can blame their enviable good figures on. The model diet goes something like this: lots of salads, lots of chicken or fish, the odd portion of rice, absolutely no bread, copious amounts of mojitos (Cuban cocktails); cigarettes instead of Pringles; and lots and lots of water. Models also dance a lot (if they're of Brazilian origin). On location, they retreat to their rooms to do yoga. At home, they exercise and go to the gym. I am sure some of them have eating disorders, just as I am sure that many do not. I know that for some a perfect figure means plastic surgery (like one 17-year-old I worked with who'd had her baby and her breast implants at the same time), and for others it's pure genetics. Models are human beings like the rest of us – it's just that sometimes they look like, well, aliens.

On the beach I make a mental note of the problems I will fix upon my return. They are as follows:

Saggy bust – only passable with Calvin Klein bra (padded and underwired for maximum support)

Bulging stomach – puffs out if it so much as sees a breadstick

Cellulite – cell-you-don't-like, actually

Pale skin – and I'm supposed to be part Asian

Hairy skin – more hairy bear than goose down

How did this all happen? Only a few years ago I didn't think twice about catching the waves on a boogy board in a little bikini on Bondi. But then I suppose childbirth, age, a sedentary office-bound lifestyle . . . the usual things I'd always read about but assumed wouldn't happen to me. Well, they came along and happened.

Look, you can't re-invent the wheel when it comes to bodies; you can only change the spare tyre. The only way to look better in a bikini is to eat less and exercise more. Sure, a tan helps, as does smooth, buffed skin, and we'll get on to those, but I'm talking about the fundamentals here.

With almost everyone around me on and off diets since they were teenagers, I thought I had done pretty well to get to thirty-four without going on one. Was it really worth embarking on a diet if it meant a lifetime of a yo-yo metabolising? But faced with Cuba and a multitude of other unveilings of my semi-naked body in broad daylight over the next few months, I figured there was no escaping it.

Michael van Straten is a nutritionist and naturopath who spent forty years helping other people to lose weight before an accident left him in need of urgent spinal surgery, for which he had to lose two stone quickly. Yet even though he has made dieting his job, he freely admits that most diets do not work for two reasons: first, most require us to reduce our calorie level to below 1500 a day. This causes the apestat – the eating equivalent of a thermostat – to go into famine mode and shut down to conserve energy. 'Until you get to starvation point your metabolism slows to match the food intake,' he explains. 'Eventually you give up in disgust, binge, and put on everything you've lost plus a few pounds, as it takes your metabolism a while to catch up with the fact that the famine is over.'

The second reason is that faddish diets – the kind that require us to give up one whole food group – carbohydrates, say, or to eat only cabbage, or only fruit before lunch, or only bananas, are all a myth. 'Quirky ideas are sexy and get lots of publicity, because no one wants to admit that the boring rules of sensible eating are the only way to succeed. Everyone wants magic bullets.' Moreover, the ones that do work can only possibly be sustained for a short-term period, to say nothing about how dangerous this can be for your health.

Besides, dieting alone won't get rid of cellulite. The best thing about cellulite – and this is really scraping the bottom of the barrel – is that it is somewhat democratic in its nature. Not globally, in that women in poor countries don't appear to worry about it (or getting that hair appointment, or the latest Prada handbag . . . but there's nothing wrong with our Western values, right?) but at least cellulite attacks everyone: fat and thin. That really is the only good thing to be said about it. Unfairly, it doesn't seem to affect men, and if it did, well, would they really care? (See p. 167.)

I really do not trust anyone or anything that claims an ability to remove cellulite permanently 'just like that'. Any approach, whether it's creams or treatments, usually requires a major commitment on behalf of the cellulite sufferer. I know what works: mesotherapy, wraps, light therapy, endermologie, but none of these are one-hit wonders, gone in an hour. Most require ten to fifteen treatments and a follow-up course a few months down the line. This represents a major commitment in both time and money, and is no easier than sticking to a regular exercise routine.

Malvina Fraser has tried them all, but has chosen to stick with light therapy. She works in a small room, just big enough to fit a massage bed, in the clinic of a cosmetic surgeon's London practice as well as in her own brand new clinic. She has gorgeous creamy skin, a mane of thick blonde hair, and a big, dazzling, sincere smile. I warm to her straight away. An accomplished facialist as well as masseur, the treatment of hers that has remained most in demand is light therapy, which uses fibre optic light that is said to penetrate to the lower layers of the skin and stimulate the circulation and eliminate toxins. The idea is that in doing this, you also get rid of cellulite.

'What do you think cellulite is caused by?' I ask her.

'Most believe it is caused by poor circulation. Which of course I do believe, because the lymph has no waste disposal system of its own, and it relies on the circulation to pop out all the toxins. And women's circulation is poor.'

'Lymph does what exactly?'

'It holds all the toxins, and if you don't get it pumped out or drink loads of water, they stay in the system. My mother is seventy-one and doesn't have so much as a centimetre of cellulite. There was no contraceptive pill years ago, and they ate good vegetables and meat. There were plenty of minerals in the soil then. Well, we're told they've all been depleted. And that's why we have to take all these supplements. Hopefully they'll be doing us some good!' she chuckles.

I have at this point undressed, and am lying face down on a massage bed, covered loosely by a blanket. Fraser starts the treatment by covering the area of my skin she is about to 'probe' (that being the fibre optic tool she uses) with a liquid gel that reacts with the probe to heat up the lower layers of the skin and get the circulation going.

'I sometimes think if cellulite appears outwardly on our skin as a result of toxins, what on earth are these toxins doing to the insides of our bodies?' I say.

'Yes. It's scary. It is very worrying,' says Fraser, not looking very scared at all, as she is still smiling at me. She turns up the dial on the little machine by the bed. 'All the drinking and eating too many dairy products, drinking coffee . . . Milk is fat, and coffee is toxins, and it depends how much of each you have. But I don't think you should deprive yourself of everything, because then you just get depressed.'

She turns on the red light and pushes the fibre-optic probe – a small fish-tail-shaped rod – up either side of my spine. I don't have cellulite in my spine,

I think, but then I remember that there is a lot of lymph concentrated in this area, which of course then goes all round the body. The machine has a whole rainbow of different-coloured lights: red, green, blue, yellow and orange, which are used according to whatever treatment Fraser is doing.

'Red is best for circulation,' she says. 'It penetrates the deepest, right down to the base of the skin. It pushes the oxygen around and helps to eliminate toxins. I usually use red quite a lot for the first few treatments, because most women's circulation is poor. And then I start to work specifically on the lymph with the lilac light. But you know, I don't think anyone can get rid of their cellulite 100 per cent. It depends a lot on your age and your lifestyle.

'Is it something you can prevent?' I ask.

'Oh yes. There are lots of models who come in specifically to keep their circulation going.'

'Which ones?'

'I can't say . . . but there's definitely no point in waiting until you get cellulite because then it just takes longer to get rid of . . . And you have to do things at home, as well.'

'Like what?

Fraser is by now working up my thighs, pushing the light in a kneading motion. It doesn't feel particularly hot – apparently the hotter it feels, the more efficient your circulation, which doesn't say much for mine. It is so gentle and painless that, combined with her calm, friendly voice, I feel myself being lulled into sleep. 'Skin brushes are very good. Even using Epsom Salts in the bath. You don't have to buy the expensive ones. It's around £5 for three kilos, and you put a cup and a half of it in the bath twice a week, and sit in it for 20 minutes. It really speeds up the circulation. You keep the water quite hot, and when you come out you should wrap up warm and drink lots of water. You just sit peacefully afterwards, otherwise you'll feel a bit dizzy. And it's not a good thing to do if you suffer from low or high blood pressure. It really works. And it's cheap.'

'What other things help with cellulite?'

'Drinking lots of water is one of the most important things you can do. Your lungs alone need a litre a day. If your lungs aren't functioning properly you're not getting the oxygen around the body.'

Fraser continues working the fibre optic up and over my body, using an accelerating motion to help speed up the circulation, and pushing it in the direction of the heart. I don't feel hot, just sleepy. I am now so relaxed I am not really listening any more.

Skin brushing. She did say *skin brushing*. One of the cheapest yet most effective remedies against cellulite, and do I ever do it? No. I forget. And yet it's so easy. You use a stiff-bristled brush, a gentle loofah, or even, if your skin is really sensitive, a natural sponge. All you do is stand in the bath or shower, and before you even turn on the tap, you brush your body upwards from toe to head, moving all the time in the direction of the heart. It takes all of five minutes. Then you shower as usual. So why don't I do it, I wonder?

As for anti-cellulite creams, Malvina Fraser has tried every product on the market and listened to her numerous well-heeled clients talk of all the products they have also tried, and she has come to the old conclusion that no cream will rid us of our cellulite in one fell swoop, unless we adhere to a healthy diet and exercise programme as well. 'Sure, they get excited at the beginning when they're trying out something new,' she says, of her clients, 'but well, this is my job and I really enjoy it, and I am not just doing this to make money. I am doing this to see results.'

I believe her. I fall asleep. I wish I could say that when I woke up all my cellulite had gone, but it hadn't. But just six treatments later, there was definitely an improvement. And what a painless, pleasurable way to do it.

HOW TO MAKE A GOOD MOJITO

This has nothing whatsoever in it to help you lose weight. It won't improve your cellulite. But some models drink quite a few when they're shooting in Cuba, and with this tenuous link in mind, I felt it was a good excuse to include something that is about sheer enjoyment. From the bar at Claridge's, this is how you do it:

In a glass put mint, sugar to taste and the juice of half a fresh lime. Add crushed ice and top with 50 ml (2 fl oz) of Havana Club (three-year-old) rum. Stir. Drink.

DRINKS THAT ARE A LITTLE HEALTHIER FOR YOU

Michael van Straten created these so that, should you be dieting, you'll get an extra kick of vitality.

BLUE PASSION

A juice guaranteed to chase away the blues and bring a glow to your skin. This tonic in a glass will give you instant energy and super immunity. Blend 100 g (4 oz) blueberries, 2 passion fruit, 1 medium cantaloupe melon and 1 mango.

SCARBOROUGH FAIR

A combination of vital force and calming influences, blend 4 carrots, 3 sticks of celery, a handful of parsley, 6 sage leaves, 2 teaspoons of rosemary (leaves removed from the stalk) and a small sprig of thyme.

BEET TREAT

This juice builds healthier blood and provides essential ingredients for cell protection. Blend 1 small beetroot, including its leaves, together with 3 carrots and 2 apples.

CELLULITE: AND NOW THE SCIENCE . . .

Actually there's very little science on cellulite. I hate to bang on about this men's versus women's bodies thing, but if men had it, you can bet they would have invented a cure for it, or at least tried to understand it. Of course, the reason they don't have it is because they don't produce oestrogen, the female hormone that keeps cellulite a purely female phenomenon.

What exactly is cellulite?

Cellulite starts with bad circulation in certain areas of the body some four to eight years before you see it. Because the circulation is poor, the wastes, fluids and toxins that normally speed around your system come to a halt in those areas. The cells don't get fed properly because nourishment can't get to them. The lymphatic system can't operate as it usually does because the tissues and fluids build up around the new blockage. If there is too much fat in the fat cells, this makes things even worse. They become engorged with fat and waste products, and hard lumps of collagen form around the cells. These then gradually harden further, leaving a nasty, lumpy old mess of sagging skin. If your hormones are all over the place, you will doubtless be storing more fat in these cells, which also causes the cells to bulge, pulling down the connective fibres that normally keep skin looking tight and firm. I'm sorry, but you did ask.

Am I a candidate for light therapy?

Yes, if your cellulite bothers you and you can afford the time and money for a full course of treatments. Yes, if you want your skin to feel super-soft – one of the side effects of speeding up circulation is that it also speeds up cell renewal, bringing new cells to the surface. No, if you are epileptic, or have had cancer or chemotherapy in the last year. Inform the therapist of these and any other serious ailments, and tell her if you are pregnant.

OTHER THINGS TO TRY

Endermologie A skin folding and rolling technique developed in France ten years or so ago. It uses a hand-held machine to 'suck' up the skin in much the same way your vacuum cleaner does when it's going over a rug as opposed to a carpet – only this time the machine keeps moving and your skin gets spat out again. It's another way to get the circulation going, the only side effect being that if you have skin that bruises easily you're liable to look a little black and blue a few days after your treatment. Otherwise, it does work, albeit temporarily, but again, commitment is key: you'll need to go twice a week for fifty minutes at a time, for a minimum of sixteen treatments before you'll see a result, and monthly maintenance after that is also required.

Mesotherapy This is an Italian medical-style treatment that involves injecting a cocktail of antioxidants, vitamin B_1 and usually sea minerals to affected areas to break down the fat and speed up the metabolism. It is painful, but promises a 90 per cent improvement in the affected areas. You will need to take a course of eight treatments, with top-up sessions to follow.

Wrap treatments Cellophane, foil, heated blankets . . . there is a wide range of treatments involving wraps that can be effective for short-term cellulite removal. Usually a mask is applied to the body, following skin brushing. The wraps cause the body to perspire, so water is lost, and you may feel thirsty afterwards and look and feel lighter due to water loss.

Ginger cure

There is a traditional Japanese remedy for cellulite which goes something like this: take a large ginger root and grate it. Squeeze the juice through muslin and dip your body brush into it for scrubbing. Make sure the brush is warm and moist before you put the ginger juice on it. Scrub your body while the skin is still dry so that the ginger stimulates the circulation. This is not such a good idea if your skin is sensitive.

CELLULITE-OLOGY: WHAT TYPE DO YOU HAVE?

Hard cellulite This is the kind you see all the time.
Soft cellulite This is the kind you see when you squeeze your skin: orange

peel skin, dimples – you know the score. The best thing I've heard it called is 'quilting' by Wendy Lewis, the beauty consultant. And just in case we're at all confused, she adds, 'And I don't mean the kind on Chanel bags.'

So you can fix the cellulite, but what about the bust?

There are no treatments or products that to my knowledge will radically and permanently re-shape and lift the bust, short of plastic surgery. However, some friends report successes with CACI, a system that promises muscle 're-education' by mimicking the body's own bioelectrical field with micro-electrical impulses delivered through metal applicators. You can expect a lift of half an inch, but you'll need a course of ten treatments plus a maintenance session once a month.

The phone rings in my hotel room in New York.

'Hi! Is that room 1609?'

'Yes,' I say, not recognising the voice.

'Hi, my name is John D. Michaels, and I'm calling to schedule a time for the massage that was booked for you.'

'What massage? Are you sure you have the right room?'

'1609, that's the one! It was booked for you as a surprise gift.'

This is a surprise all right, it's 8.45 am. Still, it's not totally inconceivable that someone – perhaps a public relations beauty person who knows I'm in town – could have done this for me. It is a little odd though.

John D. Michaels continues his spiel. 'The massage has already been paid for, but unfortunately I didn't catch the name of the person who booked it for you – they paged me.'

'Oh. Well, this is very strange . . . what kind of massage is it?'

'Well, madam, I come to your room with oils and candles, and you can have any kind of massage you want: shiatsu, tantric . . . Tips and gratuities are of course up to you.'

'Tantric?'

'. . . but whatever you choose, relaxation is guaranteed . . .'

'Tantric?!' I can't help laughing. Last time I read about tantric it was a form of sexual yoga, designed to encourage a man to delay his moment of pleasure (if you'll excuse me).

'Yes madam. I am five foot eight, white Caucasian, with brown curly hair . . .'

'Listen,' I say, laughing, 'I really don't think you have the right room, but thanks anyway . . .'

Well, they're obviously all at in New York, unlike us prudish Brits. They even have their own show about it: *Sex and the City*. It seems appropriate that my 'personal masseur' should have called this morning, as today's the day I take my life into my hands and visit the shrine of all bikini waxes: the J Sisters.

If you haven't heard of the J Sisters by now, you're probably still wearing one of those swimsuits with little modesty skirts attached. I don't know why, but a few years ago, something happened in the usually dull world of the bikini wax. A small salon near Central Park, owned and run by seven Brazilian sisters, achieved a notoriety based solely on the ability of the sisters to remove any shred of pubic hair from their clients. How did this happen? They stripped off all or most of the hair in the bikini area, their clients loved it, beauty editors heard about it, celebrities endorsed it, and, hey presto, they had a cult following that went far beyond cult. The Brazilian wax is now asked for the world over – except in Brazil, of course, where it's just a normal wax – a short back and sides I suppose.

The salon itself is curious. Flanked by huge department stores and office blocks, you enter the Vanderbilt townhouse by a tiny door and walk down a corridor that borders on shabby, up in a big clanking elevator you think you might never get out of. It is a Saturday morning, probably one of their busiest days. The receptionist greets me and shows me where to hang my coat. There is a tiny loo the size of a cupboard on one side, and lots of marble, gilding and mirrors everywhere else. It's a million miles away from the slick, modernist beauty salons of today, and utterly different from the serene order of the Elizabeth Arden Red Door day spas. I can immediately understand why the first bikini wax pioneers – those people who came here before the reviews and the celebs – would have felt they had stumbled on something unique. There is that general sense of efficiency being maintained somehow through complete chaos, and while I sit down to have my nails done, I can't help but notice how the clientele – a mix of up-town, well-to-do society ladies, younger women, fashionably dressed, and a couple of tourists from Germany (which puts paid to the myth that German women are all furry) – are all looking relaxed, smiling benignly in total acceptance of whatever will happen next.

Which is just as well, because when it does happen, it bloody hurts. After the manicure, I am shown to a seat at the back of the salon. Everyone sits comfortably flicking through the glossies, but all eyes flit to and from the two white cubicles at the end. Are they soundproofed? I wonder, as I can't hear much screaming. A client, who looks Brazilian herself, comes out of one. She is wearing impossibly tight trousers, her hair is dyed blonde, her skin is tanned, and her lips are pale pink with a darker lip line (my pet hate, incidentally). She looks great, flashy, but fun rather than tarty, and she looks like she has fun with that bikini line. I'm in next.

Okay, here goes. You lie on your back on a massage bed with your jeans, tights, knickers – everything from the waist down removed. It's a massage bed in name only. Joyce dusts you with powder and asks whether you want *everything* off, or whether she should leave a 'landing strip'. If you're at all like me you will probably start giggling hysterically – which is better than crying, I suppose. She grabs you by the ankles, and lifts them towards your face, as if changing a nappy on baby. She pours hot wax on to your nether regions (yes, YOU READ THIS RIGHT), puts a muslin cloth on top, presses it down, and then RIP!!! Up it comes, hairs and all. The ripping bit happens over and over until finally it's done. It's not the most dignified of procedures, and in terms of pain, it is definitely up there with childbirth, and in a sense the results are almost the same – one leaves you with a baby, the other leaves you as soft as a baby. It's all a little odd actually, and I feel and look a little peculiar. But still, Gwyneth Paltrow has it done all the time – her signed photo is on the wall to prove it, complete with the line, 'You changed my life.' I'm a little intrigued by this. How? How can a bikini wax possibly change someone's *life*? What is she doing with this bikini wax? Where am I going wrong? Cindy Crawford, Christy Turlington, Naomi Campbell . . . they've all got their photos on the wall too, although they don't testify to it having changed their lives. Maybe they've got something better; an eyebrow plucker or a manicurist, or, God forbid, a baby or a career. But let's not pick on Gwyneth.

Upstairs, in a small, cluttered office, I have a chat with Jonice. Only five of the seven sisters are now working; two are semi-retired. They all worked together, even as children. Jonice started, aged 11, in a salon in Brazil, but then two of them decided twenty years ago to come to New York.

'Everything was different – Brazil, the culture of the beauty salon is totally different because it's summer all year long,' Jonice says. I tell her of my son's former nanny, Sahmylle Portela, a Brazilian, who, when I was packing for a trip to Canoa Quebrada in the northern part of Brazil, burst out laughing at the sight of my bikini. To me, it was just an average-sized bikini. To her, it might as well have been a pair of Bermuda shorts. 'You know,' says Jonice, people look at you there with this big sort of bikini exactly like they look at you here with a very small bikini. They can tell you're not from here.'

The two sisters found working in New York frustrating at first; the clients seemed to be rushed in and out of appointments far too quickly for them to get to know them, or to do the job properly. They wanted to take their time with the clients but instead they were told to hurry up. 'After fighting like this, we said, "Let's open our own place", so, fifteen years ago, we offered manicures only, no bikini waxing. Seven years later, we introduced the Brazilian wax. We had a very high-class clientele who became our friends. They helped us. After a few times of a client coming here, I'd say, "I have something that I want to show you. Can I try?"'

Can you imagine after getting your manicures with your lovely therapist for months on end suddenly having the life ripped out of you with a wax? That's a quantum leap in beauty terms, surely? Apparently not, because, according to Jonice – and her present business with waxing would back this up – they loved it. 'They went home. Their husband said, "That's great," and they told their friends . . . Then the beauty editors heard about it, and then it just went crazy.'

The salon had to get press-savvy. They now have a press kit complete with a CD-Rom of magazine articles that have been written about them, pictures of Gwyneth *et al.*, photos of the salon, you name it. *Playboy* came one day and tried to call it 'the *Playboy* wax' but Jonice stuck to her guns and insisted it remained the Brazilian.

'This is not some porn thing. It's not *Playboy*, it's something from our culture. I have to be careful – no men are allowed into the salon for this reason. You should hear the questions I get asked. 'Is it called the Brazilian wax because you think Brazilians are better than Americans?' This is not what we're talking about. But it's fun. On Valentine's Day men call up and order gift vouchers for their wives . . . Some people even ask me if they can get shapes done, and if it's Valentine's Day, we will do hearts. But normally, no. We prefer not to.'

It must be hard working as a family, I think. 'I've never known it any other way. Sometimes we argue. We work together all day, every day. And sometimes we see each other at the weekends because we don't have time to see our friends. But you know what? We never talk about business at the weekends, we talk about anything but business.'

So you can't make it to New York for that bikini wax. What's a girl to do?

'The most important thing about waxing is to know that the person knows how to pull the hair correctly,' says Jonice. 'It has to be pulled against the hair, always. If a waxer really knows what she's doing, she'll follow all the directions in which the hair is growing. If she doesn't you'll get ingrowing hairs. If you feel uncomfortable, it's because the person waxing doesn't have the strength. They need to be strong, because they need to be fast. You can't think about it. Sometimes you sense that the waxer feels sorry for you, they'll say, "Are you okay?" but really she can't feel

sorry for you, otherwise she won't do it fast enough. Just do it! My sister is fifty-six years old, but she can do it in five minutes. She takes sometimes up to eighty clients a day.'

How often do you need to have it done?
Usually you can leave it for four weeks, but some people can go for up to six weeks, depending on the rate of their hair growth. Unlike shaving, which strengthens hair growth, every time you pull the hair while waxing, you cauterise the blood vessels, which in turn stops the blood supply and the hair grows less.

What is the hair like that grows back?
'Softer,' says Jonice.

Are you a beauty know-it-all?
Yes, if you can name all seven of the J Sisters. They are: Jocely, Jonice, Joyce, Janea, Juracy, Jussara and Judseia.

WAXING – HOW IT'S DONE: OTILYAH ROBERTS

Otilyah Roberts has also done Gwyneth Paltrow's bikini waxing.

'I use the old, traditional methods, with a pure, hot beeswax. First you make sure the skin is clean and free of grease, with a surgical spirit type of cleanser. Then you have to make sure the skin is dry by sprinkling on some talcum powder. This acts like a cushion between the skin and the wax. It doesn't affect the movement of the hair, but at the same time it grips so it doesn't damage the skin.' With cloth strips she then pulls the hairs off, by pressing down, and then firmly detaching back against the hair.

THE DOS AND DON'TS OF WAXING

Don't go and sunbathe straight afterwards – avoid the sun for twenty-four hours. Don't be waxed if you have a rash or an irritation. 'Avoid treatments involving heat,' says Roberts. 'Some people say, "When can I have a bath?" and I say, "Just go home and have a bath!" – you can't not bath yourself for three days!'

WAXING AND WANING – WHAT'S FASHIONABLE NOW

'In the summer I do a lot of what we call the Hollywood,' says Roberts. 'It's a full monty, basically. It will be more for sexual reasons, because a boyfriend or a husband likes it. And of course, the Brazilian, for which I leave a landing strip, or a little triangle. To make a heart, I take an eyebrow pencil and work around it, then finish it with tiny stick-on Swarovski crystals.

'Sometimes people do surprise me. I had a country lady coming once who looked like Raine Spencer but twenty years older. I said to the cloakroom lady, "She's not waiting for me, is she?" I thought she must be here for an eyebrow shape, or a bit of a moustache, because older ladies sometimes get that, but no, she wanted it all removed. Apparently she's coming back again. Of course, I couldn't ask her why.

'My personal favourite is the high bikini line, so you leave a bit of hair but not so much. When you're young you can do anything. But to be honest, when you get a bit older and you're sagging here and there, it looks a little repulsive with no hair at all.'

How did you become a bikini waxer, Otilyah Roberts?
'You know, sometimes I do look at myself and think, "Otilyah, you're not such an idiot, what are you doing here?" But at the end of the day I can't stop it.'

Otilyah Roberts came from Poland, where she was born 30 km (24 miles) from the Russian border just after the war. 'I didn't see electricity until I was fourteen, and we had no running water. I used to walk barefoot all summer, and reading was my escape. Mind you, if you don't know any better, you enjoy your life, and I had a nice childhood, there was plenty of freedom. When I was about thirteen I read a book about

Marie Curie and it occurred to me that I could be famous in this way. I went to Warsaw and trained as a nurse, and then worked in Poland for seven years. I always had a talent with people. I came to London and married a South African man, and then thought, "Oh, you stupid woman, you didn't marry a Rockefeller, you have got to find a job!" I had a friend who was a beauty therapist, and she thought my nursing experience would be useful. So I applied and I started. That's how I became a beauty therapist.'

The best beauty advice Otilyah ever had

'Never, ever go to bed with make-up on. When my grown-up daughter Lara gets up in the morning her make-up is running from the night before. I have very good skin, and it's because I cleanse and moisturise no matter how drunk I am. That is the most important thing.' By the way, when she says drunk, she's talking about a long, long time ago, and not very often.

What annoys Otilyah Roberts

'I don't like it when clients tell me what to do. There is one type who comes in and is frightened that I'm going to rip everything from them. They say, "Don't put wax there; don't do that bit". I say, "Look, you've come to an expert. I'm not going to remove every part of your body, I'm only after your hair." In the summer I have a lot of new customers and it's a nightmare. They jump all the time. I'm really patient, because in this business you have to be.'

No pain, no gain

'I tell my clients, "Have a glass of whisky before you come! Or take two Nurofen before you come, that's a painkiller."

What can you do about ingrowing hairs?

Always loofah skin, and remove ingrowing hairs with tweezers. They're caused by not waxing correctly, so it might be time to find a new waxer.

Waxing for the legs: do you go above the knee?

It's as you prefer, but thigh areas get stimulated by waxing, so it's best not to if you can avoid it.

Home waxing – is there anything worse?

'In desperation, if you can't get an appointment, you will do it yourself. I know one client who can do it on her own, in an hour. I wouldn't touch it myself, although once I did try out some products and there are some strip waxes that aren't so hard to do.'

OTHER WAYS TO REMOVE HAIR

Bleaching creams: It's not just older ladies who get moustaches – I have one too, and know loads of other women who get them. I've always found a bleaching cream to be adequate for facial hair– but Kamini Vaguela, a therapist I see for eyebrow threading, warns that bleaching creams can slowly lengthen the hair. Personally, for body areas, I think bleaching is something of a hassle.

Depilatory creams: Oh, the smell of these creams wafting from the bathroom! It's a childhood memory of my big sisters when they were teenagers, that they always had these stinky creams knocking about the place. The smells have improved, and these would be a gentle way to remove hair in the bikini area for anyone not quite ready yet for the big rip.

Electrolysis: A permanent method of hair removal, electrolysis can be carried out with a small needle (which is not ideal as it can result in the formation of scar tissue) or with a probe, which is immersed in a special ionised gel. The probe transmits a galvanic current through the skin to the hair follicles, causing the root to be destroyed by the resulting chemical reaction in the follicle.

Laser: Lasers work by damaging the hair follicle with rays of intense light. It's expensive, and there are drawbacks, such as cowboy operators who promise permanent hair removal but leave the skin looking burnt. Darker skin types should try the diode laser, which has a longer wavelength. You will need a series of treatments for a bikini line or calves.

Shaving: By far the easiest and quickest method of hair removal, although the results don't last as long, and the hair feels stubbly and horrible when it grows back. Shaving is fantastic, though: you don't have to wait to have bushy calves before you remove it all, like you do with waxing, and as far as underarms go, it's the only way to do it. Keep the water warm so that the pores open; always shave while the skin is wet and go against the way the hair grows. If you're in the bath or shower, shampoo is great for working up a lather, which makes it easier. Avoid body creams with high doses of AHAs immediately afterwards, unless you like that stinging feeling.

Threading: Kamini Vaguela suggests combining threading with electrolysis as the ultimate way to remove facial hair on the upper lip permanently. The electrolysis removes the hair permanently but takes time, so while you're waiting for it to go, have the remaining hairs temporarily removed by threading. For more on threading, see pp 86–7, where I've written about it in relation to eyebrows.

WHAT IF YOU WANT A MASSAGE AND JOHN D. MICHAELS ISN'T AROUND?

Massage is important for a well-toned, relaxed body, and in the right hands and over a course of time you can make significant improvements to skin tone. There are so many different types that choosing the right one is crucial.

Aromatherapy massage Essential oils are blended according to taste and applied with much emphasis to the body's pressure points. This is a great massage to relieve stress and muscle tension, and the essential oils will increase your sense of well-being.

Ayurvedic massage Ayurveda originated in India thousands of years ago, and is a way of life, with holistic medicine and diet central to its philosophy. The Shiro Dhara is the key massage to ayurvedic treatments. Dhara means oil, and what happens is that herbal oil is dripped on to the chakras, the key energy points of the body, to restore balance and a sense of harmony. It's a pleasant treatment with swift, gentle strokes that are excellent for relaxation and skin softness, but it won't get rid of the knots in your shoulders or your cellulite.

Balinese massage If you have ever visited Bali, you will understand how important massage and a sense of well-being is to the Balinese. A typical treatment is the Lulur, a pampering ritual with an exfoliating treatment using native spices like ginger, sandalwood and turmeric, followed by a massage with long kneading strokes. You might find yogurt being used to moisturise the skin, and perhaps a bath filled with tropical flowers and essential oils will follow.

Deep-tissue massage Lots of kneading, rolling and pinching ensures that tense, stiff areas of the body are de-knotted and de-stressed. Regular treatments will help with muscle tone.

Lymph drainage massage Specialised massage movements that help decongest, detoxify and de-stress not just areas with cellulite but the whole body. It increases blood circulation to improve skin tone, and helps break down areas of subcutaneous fat. This is one of the most effective treatments you can have, and is powerful yet pampering.

Shiatsu massage A fully clothed massage that involves the masseur manipulating your limbs gently. Don't be surprised if he uses his feet to apply pressure. A good shiatsu massage will unblock energy blockages and have benefits on the mind as well as the body.

Swedish massage A more invigorating massage technique, excellent for getting rid of knots and muscle aches and pains.

Thai massage An ancient technique not dissimilar to having yoga 'performed' on you, Thai massage is given by applying pressure along the energy meridians of the body, together with stretching the muscles. You'll feel energised, tight muscles feel looser, and overall you should feel calmer and more peaceful. You are fully clothed for this massage.

Advice I have gleaned from massage therapists over the years boils down to the following

Always take all your clothes off, provided you feel comfortable, so that the therapist can work around the largest muscles of the body: the gluteals. To find a good masseur, stick with the large companies like Clarins and Decleor, who invest a lot of time and money in training their staff, or ask a friend whose opinion you respect. The gift of massage is in the hands, and you will know on first touch whether that masseur is right for you or not. At any rate, never put up with a massage if the pressure isn't hard or soft enough. Ask your therapist politely, and with any luck, they will welcome your participation. If you don't like the music, or the temperature of the room, let your therapist know straight away. If you're a man, having a massage is not a green light to make unwelcome sexual advances to your therapist.

A slip of paper, rolled and tied with straw and fastened with a tiny stone dolphin, lies on my bed. Inside is a quotation from Sir Isaac Newton: *'To myself, I seem to have been only like a boy playing on the seashore, diverting myself now and then finding a smoother pebble or a prettier shell than the ordinary, whilst the great ocean of truth lay all undiscovered before me.'* I don't know if it's an ocean of truth, but the turquoise ocean before me is certainly inspiring. The Four Seasons hotel in the Maldives invited me to review their new spa, and of course I was happy to oblige. My room, a bungalow on stilts that is more in the sea than beside the sea, has a bedroom with a glass window wall to wall, through which shimmering blues of every hue look back at me like a Dulux paint card. At the top, bright blue, where the sky meets the horizon; just below, dark blue, where the Indian Ocean is deep and dangerous; below, a thin line of white surf where the deep blue hits the coral reef; and finally, the thickest layer, glorious aqua moving like mercury in gentle, light-reflecting waves – a view that is interrupted only by the odd boat or shoal of fish swimming past.

I suppose if you insist on finding some deep parallel between the quote from Isaac Newton (quotes are the new chocolate on the pillow at bed-time) and the beauty industry, there is something there. Our distractions are the latest quick-fix beauty cures, which of course offer nothing except excitement of dubious merit at the beginning, quickly replaced by huge disappointment at one's own stupidity for falling for them. Wading through all the schnick and shnack, the universal truth is that there is no such thing as a free lunch. You have to do all these things regularly, responsibly, and if we're looking for another 'r', for the sake of it, rigorously. Then, and only then, will we see results.

Fortunately, there are some short-cuts worth taking. One I would recommend to anyone embarking on shedding the layers in favour of the bikini is the fake tan. Like waxing, it's a thing that is difficult to do yourself. Also like waxing, it is something that with our knowledge of the harm sunbathing and sunbeds can do to us, has become incredibly popular in a short space of time.

Tans are like cars – we know they're bad for us, but we're not prepared to give them up just yet. Coco Chanel was one of the first to make tanning popular – she loved the outdoors so much she made her own protective moisturiser called Crème du Jour. Despite the cautions about skin cancer we read in every May issue of every women's magazine, only the brave and the ginger among us stay away from the sun. I have always had as my trump card those Burmese genes, which lie dormant each year until summer hits, and then Boom! I am looking 'a bit foreign', as Laura, the deputy beauty editor at *Tatler* would laughingly say. Not as foreign as I used to look: even as a five-year-old, I was conscious of the effect my skin colour had on others. I remember being stopped on the street running back from the beach in Southwold, where my grandmother had a house. A stranger said, 'You look like an Indian!' I burst into tears and ran all the way back. Looking Indian was not fashionable as a five-year-old thirty years ago. My swimming teacher in Maidstone constantly referred to me as her 'little drop of sunshine', which should really be treated with the warmth and generosity of spirits with which she said it, but at the time, coming back from nearly three years of sun exposure in Malta, only served to single me out even more as the new kid from the thirty or so pale-skinned classmates.

How times have changed. The truly fashionable have the fake tan down pat. Not for them looking like a lobster, painfully inching their way towards that famous stocking shade: American Tan. Fake tans work thanks to dihydroxy-acetone (DHA), which is harmless to the skin, but reacts with the proteins and amino acids in the top layer to turn the skin a brownish colour. In the last few years, manufacturers have added lots of natural-sounding ingredients to make them feel and smell better, and there's certainly no harm in that. They used to turn you orange – the consultants at beauty counters were notorious for their orange faces and white coats – but now they're indistinguishable from the real thing.

Judy Naake had been a beauty therapist for years before an obscure tanning product was sent to her to try out. Coming from California, what made this one different was an aloe vera base, which left the skin feeling incredibly soft, and gave a deeper-coloured tan. But the really clever thing about it was the fact that when you applied it, instead of sinking into the skin, it left a muddy trace. Mud, you might think, would not be very desirable as a tan, and yet it meant you could see exactly what you were doing when you were applying it, and rinse off the muddy effect once it had been allowed to take (a few hours). There was none of that fear of having missed a bit. Naake jumped straight on a plane to LA, met the owner, and brought the product back to England, this time in bulk, and this time as its distributor.

It didn't 'happen' straight away. 'The therapists were wary of it,' Naake says, 'and didn't know how to apply it properly. I'd invested everything into this, and I couldn't afford for it to go wrong. So I embarked on a tour of Britain, and

I went and gave lectures and demonstrations on how to apply it.' Her hard work paid off, thanks also to a clever name which captured the public's imagination in a way that no other fake tan had done before. Today the St Tropez tan has gone from being something only the beauty cognoscenti – the celebs and the editors – knew about to selling at two or three million orders at a time in Boots.

'That's a lot of tan!' says Naake. 'The idea is that you can now have a treatment, and then top it up yourself when it starts to fade. Well, you can't send a client home without giving her some product, because how else will she keep it going? It's not fair to take the money off people just for a treatment, because it is not cheap, and it will begin to fade after three days.'

And her clients do do it themselves at home. Even Posh Spice. 'She does, you know. In fact she phoned last week from Manchester and asked me where she could buy it, because she hadn't any in Manchester. So she does do it herself. I struggle with mine sometimes because you need to get to the back of the ankles, and unless you've been to the gym, that is hard. Doing your back is difficult as well, which is why we've brought out a roller.'

'Is that like a roller you paint walls with?' I ask.

'Yes and no. It's long, so it fits the shape of your back.'

I can't imagine ever doing this by myself at home. It's so much nicer to lie back and have her do it for you. Naake kindly obliges, and a few hours later (the treatment takes one hour, the tan needs another three hours to develop, and it lasts about seven days) I am tanned all over. It's relaxing, but not as soothing as a massage, because, as you would expect, you have to keep lifting a leg up here, and popping an arm over there, so she can make sure she has covered you evenly. As she works her way around an armpit, I ask her how you can do this yourself, à la Posh.

'The most important thing is to exfoliate before you apply,' she says. 'That way it will last longer and go on more evenly. You need to moisturise your dry bits, like elbows and knees, and anywhere that you don't want to be so dark, like the joints of the fingers. You then have to make sure you cover the whole body, including those armpits. You must remove your deodorant before you start, otherwise it will turn green as the chemicals react, and you will look like the Incredible Hulk. Take perfumes off as well. If you want a lighter shade – for example on the face – mix the tan with some moisturiser.'

The interesting thing is that even though I am part Burmese, and expecting therefore to look orange or grey, the finished result is absolutely spot on. Two weeks in the Caribbean, no problem.

Or even better, the Maldives. Exposed as I am now to the real thing, the sun, even with a fake tan, I need protection. We all do. Back at Dr Polis's office, several black women were coming to have their moles checked. According to Cancer Research UK, skin cancer is the most common cancer in the UK, with 6000 out of an estimated 46,000 cases per year being malignant melanoma – a deadly form of the disease. Lying on the white sand watching the miniature pearly coloured crabs spin their eyes around before they scurry back into their holes, it occurs to me that I probably shouldn't even be doing this. But life is short, it is not always much fun, so hey, slip, slap, slop, put the protection on, and lie back and enjoy yourself.

What they do in hot countries

I once went on a trip to Myanmar (Burma). It is the most beautiful country in the world, even if it is incredibly poor and run by a horrendously cruel military dictatorship (that's my next entry visa gone . . .). I met my second cousins and picked up a few beauty tips from them. First I was 'fat', although this was intended as a compliment, and second, I should put some thanaka on my face. Thanaka is a paste made from the ground bark of a tree. The bark is mixed with water and then applied all over the face. It has cooling benefits and acts as a natural sunblock. I wonder if also it isn't some natural bleaching agent, as they said it would be good for my freckles. Freckles, in most Asian countries, are a big no-no.

Fake tan versus sunbed: which is the ultimate winner?

Fake, of course, or sunless tanning, as the sophisticated call it. Not only is it infi-

nitely safe, as long as you still remember you need to wear a sunscreen when you're exposing your body to the sun, but it has a better finish. 'You can tell when someone has been on a sunbed because they have white lines here and pressure points on the back and shoulder blades. Fake is also better than a sunbed because you don't have to turn over. All you have to do is cover yourself completely,' says Naake.

Sunscreen: what you need to be protected

The principle, which you will have heard a thousand times before, is that if you would normally burn in about ten minutes, wearing an SPF of 10 will give you 100 minutes of protection time; if you wear an SPF of 20 you will have 200 minutes of protection time, etc. The problem with this is that when sunscreens are tested, they apply about 30 g (1 oz) of sunscreen to the whole body. 'But in real life,' says Jane Oppenheim of Australian sunscreen company Sunsense, 'we're putting on a third of the amount they use for testing. That's why people should use high SPF products – because you're only putting a third on. You should also bear in mind that you start getting DNA damage a long time before you see the reddening in the skin. Your propensity towards skin cancers, or photo ageing, is the total accumulation of sunlight that you get through your lifetime, so living in Australia you really must wear sunscreen every day. And I would recommend most people wear it in the summer months everywhere else.'

No body hair, a fake tan, no cellulite . . . what's left to do?

Well, there is always exercise. Let's save that for another book. There's also exfoliation and moisturisation. If you're dry-skin brushing, that's all you need to do to exfoliate, and do you really need me to tell you how to slather on a moisturiser?

Conclusion
AND ANOTHER THING . . .

We live in a shallow world. More than a decade after Naomi Wolf wrote *The Beauty Myth*, the feminist polemic that investigated the impact of the beauty industry on women's lives, not much has changed. Indeed, some things probably never will – like male newscasters being haggard, their wrinkles imbuing them with a sense of wisdom and importance, while female newscasters are invariably under forty, slim, with perfect hair-dos and perfect make-up. But more frighteningly, the easy availability of anti-wrinkle remedies that actually work, plastic surgery that is more accessible than ever before, and the ascent of the celebrity icon as universal beauty queen while heralded as liberating women from the fear of looking old (oh! the shame!) have actually increased the pressures to remain young and attractive. We truly know how to be beautiful – at least according to the shallow definition imposed by society – so what's stopping us?

I think we will always be obsessed (and I use that word in the loosest sense) with looking the best we can. Of course, there are more important things to worry about, but it is not for nothing that the words 'beauty' and 'therapy' are used in conjunction with each other. For me, the truly positive thing about the beauty industry is that anything we do for ourselves in such stressful, busy times can only have a good effect. This is an arena that is exclusively our own. (Sure, men are jumping on the bandwagon, but who's interested in shaving cream and ingrowing hairs?) The pressures of trying to be all things to all people are taking their toll but we have a whole swathe of products and treatments just dying to cater to our needs. You have only to look at the massive trend for spas, home beauty services and aromatherapy in every guise to see how pampering at the smallest level has become a necessity and not a luxury.

Wolf's manifesto had the positive effect of forcing a dialogue, a discussion, and entered the psyche of women's magazine editors whether they liked it or not. Some did like – shoots were dropped where models looked too skinny, and our stereotype of a model being five foot ten with Miss World statistics gave way to allow the inclusion of different types of beauties such as the more curvaceous Sophie Dahl and the shorter Kate Moss. It was generally accepted, if not publicly acknowledged, that super-skinny models were perhaps not the best role models for impressionable young women. But some didn't like – I remember being told in the strongest terms by the female editor of one women's glossy I worked at as a junior beauty assistant, 'This is not a *feminist* magazine, you know.'

As a beauty editor, what myths would I smash today if I could?

1 **Stop this celebrity madness.** We believe too much in the beautiful people. We're surrounded by celebrity endorsements that we hate ourselves for falling for (*Gwyneth Paltrow loves MAC Spice lipstick!*). We aspire to the unattainable, from models in glossy magazines who are ten years younger and ten stone thinner to celebrity faces on hoardings selling us the latest offerings from the billion-dollar beauty industry. The availability of new technology and the discoveries from the worlds of medicine and science have given us the power to achieve the unachievable, to look like the beautiful people. But do we really want to? I don't believe that celebrities in the music and film world (who, let's face it, are often women whose lives sometimes don't stand up to much scrutiny, yet who are happy to sell their images in return for a fat cheque and some added exposure) present a more attainable role model than their predecessors, the supermodels. I no more relate to Jennifer Lopez, Catherine Zeta-Jones, or Penelope Cruz than I did to Kate Moss, Naomi Campbell or Cindy Crawford.

2. **Get rid of harmful ingredients.** One of the biggest beauty myths today is the way we are sold products that claim to be good for us, but that are in fact full of ingredients that are poisonous. In the search for the causes of cancer in Western society, we scrutinise our diets, and we question our levels of stress, but one area that in my opinion has been overlooked is the toxins we ingest trans-dermally on a daily basis. There is a huge market for a range of skincare, bath products and cosmetics for men, women and children that would exclude harmful, sometimes carcinogenic ingredients. Some of the worst offenders are:

coal tar colours (made from the liquid in bituminous coal, which can contain a number of toxins). Most of these colours have yet to be tested for safety by the FDA, and whilst some were banned in the Fifties after children became ill from digesting them in popcorn, other dyes are known to cause skin irritation, allergic reactions, contact dermatitis and tumours in laboratory animals, yet are still used in lipsticks, dandruff shampoos and other beauty products.

formaldehyde Found in nail polishes, soap and shampoos, formaldehyde has already been banned in Sweden and Japan because of the risk of lung cancer and DNA damage, but is still allowed within the EU and the USA.

sodium laureth sulfate Found in 90 per cent of all shampoos, as well as in some toothpastes and skin creams, sodium laureth sulfate is a common cause of skin sensitivity. Its only purpose is to add suds and foam, to make products seem more luxurious and appealing. Some mainstream companies have already removed it. These include Aveda, which, when Estée Lauder bought the company a few years ago, the more cynical among us wrongly assumed would be dumping its eco-awareness ideals. Far from it, the company has just replaced this toxic ingredient with babassu from Brazil.

These ingredients are just the tip of the iceberg and more research is definitely needed. However I cannot help but find this whole area completely frightening – the beauty industry is creating products that are destined at the very least to increase our skin's sensitivity, and at the very worst, may cause cancer. Not only that, but whole ranges of 'natural' or 'organic' products are marketed as being somehow good for us, yet sometimes are the worst offenders. How cynical is that? How offensive is that? How mysoginistic is that?

3 **Give us products we really need.** Skincare giants are under duress to persuade women to part with their hard-earned cash to buy yet more products they don't actually need. Now there's nothing wrong with that – it's called capitalism. But perhaps the industry needs to be a little more imaginative with the products it sees. Time and again throughout the interviews I did for this book, the experts I talked to complained of a lack of originality. I would add to that a lack of individuality, a lack of freshness, a lack of imagination. Let's have perfumes that make our hearts sing and aren't just churned out to fulfil a yearly quota; let's have skincare that is fresh and free of harmful chemicals and not a gimmicky product to phase out other products that are no longer so marketable; let's have campaign 'faces' who will speak without being censored, who will say something interesting instead of a cute advertising soundbite. Risk-takers in business are often the ones who succeed. Let's take some risks!

4 **Give us advertising that doesn't promise miracles, or worse still, patronise us.** Now don't get me wrong. Things are changing. We're not at the stage yet where we can throw that pinch of salt over our shoulder instead of taking it with every advertisement we see, but at least things have become a little more real.

As an example of how things have improved, Robin Derrick, the art director of British *Vogue*, told me a great story about one anti-ageing skincare campaign he worked on in the Eighties: 'The line above the cream was,

'The secret of eternal youth.' I remember saying to the big boss, whose name I luckily can't remember, 'You can't get away with saying that! Nobody will believe you!' and he said, 'Of course, women won't believe it. But the great thing is, they'll do it anyway.'

Well, shock horror, women won't do it anyway. This may come as a shock to the advertising industry, but we know that rubbing a cream on our backsides is not going to get rid of cellulite overnight, after fourteen nights, or after 300 nights. We're prepared to accept it will make our skin look and feel smoother. But get rid of cellulite? Come on.

And please stop trying to outdo each other with pseudo-scientific claims about percentages of added moisturisation/wrinkle disappearance/life enhancement. The competition between one product's claim (68 per cent more moisture) and another's (70 per cent more moisture) is a huge turn-off. And, by the way, we know that putting on a lipstick might change our mood – but it's not going to change our lives.

5 **Hold the retouching.** Retouching – the changes made by computer that enhance a photograph during post-production – has become part and parcel of every photographic shoot, and is no more 'cheating' than a photographer using light creatively to enhance a model's bone structure. But in my opinion, a little bit of reality once in a while never did anyone any harm. I accept that we want images that take us away from the humdrum reality of everyday wardrobe despair, ugly face day, or bad hair week, but I question the art in taking it to such extremes that we don't even give reality a passing nod of approval. How much is too much? Once, shooting a story about plastic surgery, I asked the make-up artist why he wasn't putting any foundation and concealer on the model's slightly spotty skin. 'Oh, I'm not going to bother,' he said. 'The lipstick's the main thing. And the photographer makes her skin look so perfect after retouching that there's no point.'

I tried to turn what I perceived to be a negative into a positive.

'That's amazing,' I said. 'Imagine, maybe models won't be redundant after twenty-one years of age. We can retouch their wrinkles a little and just keep their amazing bone structure.'

'Oh, I wouldn't go that far . . .'

Call me a Luddite, but I'd say if our obsession with retouching continues the way it is, we won't even need make-up artists in the near future.

6 Sisters are doing it to themselves. Finally, can we just be a bit nicer to each other about the way we look? For all I joke about my husband laughing at my fat post-baby tummy, it is we women who are sometimes our own worst enemies. We are super-critical about our images, constantly self-deprecating, and while this sometimes has disastrous consequences – anorexia and bulimia to name just two – it has a lesser, but still serious, trickle-down effect on our psyche. I wrote this book not because I thought that we should all somehow transform ourselves into being beautiful beings, but because we are already beautiful creatures and we deserve to celebrate that. And no, your bum doesn't look big in that. Well, okay, just a little.

None of these things will bring us the world peace that many a beauty queen has craved, but they will make a difference to our perception of ourselves, and bring an improvement to our lives. And that's more than can be said for Hope in a Jar. Because the true answer to how to be beautiful is something we know. We have it already. Inside.

USEFUL RESOURCES

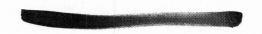

The following are contactable for further information:

John Barrett (and William Howe)
John Barrett Salon,
754 5th Avenue,
NY 10019, New York, USA
Tel: 001 212 872 2700
www.johnbarrett.com

Bastien Gonzales
Claridges,
Olympus Health and Fitness Suite,
Brook Street,
London W1A 2JQ
Tel: 020 7629 8860

Home House,
20 Portman Square,
London W1H 9HF
Tel: 020 7670 2000

Hôtel Bristol,
108 rue du Fbg St-Honoré,
Paris 75008
Tel: 00 331 42 66 24 22

Hôtel Costes,
239 rue Saint-Honoré,
Paris 75001
Tel: 00 331 42 44 50 35

www.bastiengonzales.com

Nicky Clarke
Flagship salon: Nicky Clarke Mayfair,

130 Mount Street,
London W1K 3NY
Tel: 020 7491 4700

Nicky Clarke Manchester
Unit A, 16 The Triangle,
Exchange Square,
Manchester M4 3TR
Tel: 0161 833 3555

Products available at Boots and Pure
Beauty

For free haircare advice and product
information call 0845 6014634
www.nickyclarke.com

Barbara Daly
c/o Dowal Walker PR,
Unit 13.1.1, The Leather Market,
Weston Street,
London SE1 3ER
Tel: 020 7378 7817

Make-up range available at larger
branches of Tesco
For nearest branch call 0800 505 5555

Terry de Gunzberg
10 Avenue Victor Hugo,
Paris 75016
Tel: 00 331 44 76 00 76
www.byterry.com

Roja Dove
For perfume consultations and
bespoke perfume call 01273 383458
email: r.dove@rdprgroup.com

Malvina Fraser
25 Wimpole Street,
London W1G 86L
Tel: 020 7637 0548

57 Poland Street,
London W1F 7NW
Tel: 020 7439 2895

www.malvina-beauty.com

John Frieda
4 Alford Street,
London W1Y 5PU
Tel: 020 7491 0840

75 New Cavendish Street,
London W1N 7RB
Tel: 020 7636 1401

Claridges,
Brook Street,
London W1K 4HR
Tel: 020 7499 3617

797 Madison Avenue,
New York, NY 10021, USA
Tel: 001 212 879 1000

Sally Hershberger @ John Frieda
8440 Melrose Place, Los Angeles, CA
90069, USA
Tel: 001 323 653 4040

John Frieda
030 East 76th Street
New York, NY 10021, USA
Tel: 001 212 327 3400

Products available at John Frieda
Salons, Boots, Tescos and Superdrug

www.johnfrieda.com

Daniel Galvin
42–44 George Street,
London W1U 7ES
For stocklists call 020 7486 8601
www.daniel-galvin.co.uk

Peter Gray
Represented by Untitled Management,
72 Wardour Street,
London W1F OTD
Tel: 020 7434 3202

Hamilton
Represented by Shine,
3M Cooper House,
2 Michael Road,
London SW6 2AD
Tel: 020 7736 8310
www.shinestyling.com

Lyn Harris
Miller Harris,
14 Needham Road,
London W11 2RP
Tel: 020 7221 1545

For mail order and stockists
call 020 7620 1771

J Sisters
35 West 57th Street,
New York, NY 10019, USA
Tel: 001 212 750 2485
www.jsisters.com

Philip Kingsley
54 Green Street,
London W1K 6RU
Tel: 020 7629 4004

16 E 53rd Street, New York

NY 10022, USA
Tel: 001 212 753 9600

For stockists call 020 7629 4004
www.philipkingsley.co.uk

Wendy Lewis & Co
210 East 79th Street,
New York, NY 10021, USA
Tel: 001 212861 6148

15 Sloane Gardens,
London SW1W 8EB
Tel: 0870 743 0544

www.wlbeauty.com

Eve Lom
2 Spanish Place,
London W1U 3HU
Tel: 020 7935 9988

For mail order call 020 8773 3990
For Eve Lom facials nationwide
call 020 7935 9988

Sam McKnight
Represented by Premier,
1st Floor,
7–8 St. Stephen's Mews,
London W2 5Q3
Tel: 020 7221 2333

Dr Daniel Maes
c/o Estée Lauder Press Office,
Estee Lauder,
73 Grosvenor Street,
London W1K 3BQ
Tel: 020 7409 6822

For stockists or customer information
call 01730 232566
www.esteelauder.com

Dr Danné Montagu-King
Flagship Clinic,
117A Harley Street,
London W1G 6AT

For stockists or customer information
call 0151 348 4490

DMK Skin Revision Center,
415 North Crescent Drive,
Suite 220, Beverly Hills,
CA 90210, USA
Tel: 001 310 275 7295

www.dannemking.com

Kay Montano
Represented by Streeters,
Room 504 A,
568 Broadway,
New York,
NY 10012, USA
Tel: 001 212 219 9566

Jade Moon at Michaeljohn
Michaeljohn,
25 Albemarle Street,
London W1S 4HU
Tel: 020 7629 6969
www.salonspa.co.uk

Jackie Denholm Moore
at Les Senteurs,
71 Elizabeth Street,
London SW1W 9PJ
Tel: 020 7730 2322

Judy Naake
St Tropez Beauty Source,
72 Windsor Street,
Beeston,
Nottingham NG9 LBW
Tel: 0115 922 1462
www.st-tropez.co.uk

Products available at House of Fraser,
Selfridges and Boots
www.st-tropez.com

Marian Newman
c/o Mark Smith at MRA,
10 Woodman Works
204 Durnsford Road,
London SW19 8DR
Tel: 020 8971 2000

Phytologie
6 Bankside Building,
9 Risborough Street,
London SE1 OHS.
For stockist information and treatment details call 020 7620 1771
www.phytologie.com

Dr Laurie Polis
SoHo Integrated Health Center,
62 Crosby Street,
New York, NY 10012, USA
Tel: 001 212 431 1600
www.sohoderm.com

Otilyah Roberts
Otilyah Roberts at Daniel Hersheson
45 Conduit Street,
London W1S 2YN
Tel: 020 7434 1747

Linda Rose
For stockists call 001 800 937 9146
www.lindarose.com

Glauca Rossi
10 Sutherland Avenue,
London W9 2HQ

For courses and cosmetics
call 020 7289 7485
www.glaucarossi.com

Eugene Soulieman
Represented by Streeters,
2–4 Old Street, London EC1V 9AA
Tel: 020 7253 3949

Sunsense (Jane Oppenheim)
32 Canon Street,
St. Albans AL3 5JS
stephaniespencer@yahoo.com
Tel: 01727 847480

For stockist information
call 00 35316 20 40000

Charlotte Tilbury
Represented by Untitled,
72 Wardour Street,
London W1F OTD
Tel: 020 7434 3202
www.untitled.uk.com

Christy Turlington
c/o Sundari
379 West Broadway,
Suite 404, New York,
NY 10012, USA

For Sundari skincare stockists
call 020 7235 5000
www.sundari.com

Kamini Vaguela
15 Wyndham Place,
London W1H 1AQ
Tel: 020 7723 8838,
020 8643 3268

Michael van Straten
Glebe House,
Station Road,
Chettington,
Leighton Buzzard,
Bedfordshire LU7 OSG
Tel: 01296 661215

Charles Worthington

Charles Worthington,
7 Percy Street,
London W1P 9FB
Tel: 020 7631 1370

34 Great Queen Street,
London WC2B 5AA
Tel: 020 7831 5303

The Broadgate Club,
1 Exchange Place,
London EC2M 2QT
Tel: 020 7638 0802

Triton Square,
Regents Place,
London NW1 3XB
Tel: 020 7383 4840

The Dorchester,
Park Lane,
London W1A 2HJ
Tel: 020 7317 6321

Products available at Charles
Worthington Salons and Boots
www.cwlondon.com

INDEX